Sacroiliac Joint Pain
For Tens of Thousands the Pain Ends Here

Author

BRUCE E DALL, MD

Forward by

MICHAEL R MOORE, MD

DallHouse Productions
Kalamazoo, Michigan
Sijointpaingone.com

The author is grateful to the following entities for allowing use of copyrighted material:
Springer Publishing; 5 images
Borgess Health Alliance; Appendix One Algorithm
ZYGA Corp; Appendix Two Algorithm

Cover Design by
River Run Press, Kalamazoo, MI

First Edition

ISBN: 978-0-9993804-4-4 (River Run Press)
ISBN: 978-0-9993804-8-2 (Createspace)
ISBN: 978-0-9993804-5-1 (Kindle)
ISBN: 978-0-9993804-3-7 (audio)

This book is dedicated to

All the patients that taught me so much about
Sacroiliac Joint Pain

Table of Contents

Appendix Two

Contains the Algorithm to educate surgeons on an appropriate method for patient rehabilitation after a lateral minimally invasive sacroiliac joint fusion.

Forward

Many people believe that medicine makes progress in a steady fashion, with the state of medical knowledge ever improving and the tools available to doctors advancing in a positive direction by the day, if not by the hour. The truth is that medical progress frequently does not advance in this way. Surprising to many, there are times when even in the modern era, the state of knowledge not only does not progress, but also actually slides backwards. Such was the case in the 20th Century with regard to the sacroiliac joint and its role in low back pain. Dr. Dall's book illuminates the story of how, prior to the 1930's, even with little of the technology we take for granted today, most physicians treating low back pain were aware that the sacroiliac joint could be the culprit in many patients and directed what treatment tools they had toward the sacroiliac joint as the source. Paradoxically, advances in x-ray technology that allowed the discovery of other causes of low back pain and sciatica led physicians to forget the role of the sacroiliac joint as a cause of low back pain nearly altogether. By the time the generation of physicians of which Dr. Dall and I are both members were being educated, the sacroiliac joint had been completely eliminated from any discussion of low back pain. Any question a young medical student or resident might bring up regarding the possible role of the sacroiliac joint as a cause of low back pain was met with derision and an implied or explicit admonishment not to bring it up again.

There is a hubris that exists in all eras that inclines the belief that we have finally reached a point where mistakes of the past will not be made again. We chuckle at how people could have at one time believed the Earth was flat, or that all of the planets and stars moved around a stationary Earth. Dr. Dall tells the modern day story of how the sacroiliac joint, which is now known to be the cause of perhaps one out of every five cases of one of the most common human maladies, was neglected for the most of the 20th century, and remains neglected by a significant portion of the medical community in the 21st Century. He takes us through his personal journey of the rediscovery of the sacroiliac joint as a cause of low back pain, and illustrates the human consequences of modern medicine's failure to remember what it had already learned. Patients came to him after being told, "nothing could be done." Real patients, with real problems, had been robbed of hope. Fortunately for them, they had found their way to a rebel physician who had insisted on exploring the truth and who ignored the institutional and peer pressure that existed at the time.

Dr. Dall is eminently qualified to author this book. Among the handful of us who believed the sacroiliac joint caused pain and that this pain could be treated, he was the first to successfully publish his results and findings in a respected research journal. This must be considered a major accomplishment. Physicians who occupy positions such as editors of research journals and Directors of residency programs are people who have worked in academic medicine and built reputations over decades. Such people are not easily persuaded to new ideas, especially when the ideas originate outside of the University. I recall receiving a particularly critical rejection of a paper I had submitted to a journal from the Editor-in-Chief, a famous and highly respected surgeon, who suggested I not submit any similar material in the future. This particular surgeon had authored a popular book on low back pain, in which there was no mention of the sacroiliac joint whatsoever. One can imagine how difficult it would be for someone who had achieved worldwide fame as an expert on low back pain to accept the notion that there was an entire group of patients that he or she had either misdiagnosed or ignored throughout his or her entire career. That Dr. Dall was able to overcome this type of prejudice, which was pervasive at the time, is a testament to his persistence, tenacity, and devotion to helping patients as well as to bringing the truth to light.

Dr. Dall also reveals the rarely discussed idea that all encounters between a physician and a patient are two-way human interactions. The patient arrives with the expectation that they will learn something from the physician. A good physician will also learn something from every patient encounter. Dr. Dall is singularly honest in his description of interactions with particular patients in which he admits to uncertainty and not having answers immediately at hand. Doctors are taught to portray a persona who has all the answers at their fingertips in any situation. The fact is that complicated problems often require complicated solutions. Even the most brilliant mathematician cannot solve difficult problems without some time to think about them. Patients for whom there was no established treatment came to Dr. Dall. One could not look up how to treat someone with a sacroiliac problem, as the textbooks of the time did not even acknowledge the existence of the diagnosis, much less describe a treatment algorithm. He was willing to abandon the scripted persona of having all the answers immediately and he was forthright in telling his patients he would have to give their problem some serious thought. As the book describes, patients were understanding of his approach and the results were ultimately positive.

The context of the environment in which Dr. Dall undertook his personal exploration is important to consider. The United States is among the most litigious countries on the planet. It requires significant courage for a surgeon to undertake a novel operation on a patient for a condition, which is in itself controversial. He risks lawsuits, loss of reputation, and even possibly loss of his medical license if results are not as desired and the case is reviewed unfavorably. I recall being at a national research meeting in the 1990's when the subject of SI fusions was under discussion. In front of an audience that included several hundred spine surgeons, a prominent academic surgeon stood up and said he would personally testify against any surgeon who was sued for performing an elective SI fusion. I suspect that surgeon now hopes no one remembers his blanket statement. In one of life's amusing ironies, this same surgeon subsequently published at least one article relating to the surgical treatment of sacroiliac joint dysfunction.

Dr. Dall has placed a very human face on a real medical problem that has for too long been ignored and under treated. Pendulums tend to swing, and he also points out the need for accurate diagnosis as the danger exists that as more physicians become aware of the problem, there may be patients who are erroneously treated for sacroiliac problems when the actual problem lies elsewhere. My hope is that this book will find its way both to patients with sacroiliac problems and to the physicians who care for them. Dr. Dall has played a significant role in getting the medical world back on track after losing its way for nearly 90 years.

Michael R Moore, MD
Emeritus Surgeon, The Bone & Joint Center, Bismarck, North Dakota
Spine Surgery Consultant, Phoenix, Arizona

Preface

At one time or another, 80% of Americans are affected by back pain, with the majority feeling it in their low backs

My passion to understand how the chronically painful sacroiliac joint relates to many back problems began in the early 1990s, when I was practicing at Borgess Medical Center, and encountered my first patient, Joan, with this precise diagnosis. I realized that despite all my years of training, none of it addressed Joan's chronic pain problem. Although the medical system had a lot to say about acute sacroiliac joint pain from trauma (i.e. auto accident) and infection, it had really nothing to offer a doctor, to include surgeons, for effectively treating chronic disabling sacroiliac joint pain. As I began to study and research the intricacies of the sacroiliac joint, I discovered that there were only a handful of spinal surgeons in the country who really understood this condition and had ideas on how to approach treatment, most of which had been learned through self-training.

Joan's case led me to make a conscious decision to learn all I could about chronic pain stemming from the sacroiliac joint. Once I began earnestly looking for it, I soon found dozens of patients appearing to be suffering from pain due to this joint. Since I had been taught to definitively diagnose other areas of back pain with injections, I began to inject my patients with a pain-numbing anesthetic to confirm the diagnosis of sacroiliac joint pain. Over the years, this injection technique has been refined by pain management doctors, and has now become the standard for accurately diagnosing this condition. Then, using modifications of the surgery I had first created for Joan, I performed several more sacroiliac fusions on people who had experienced no relief from existing conservative treatments, such as chiropractic manipulation, wearing a circular band or brace around the area of the sacroiliac joints, formal physical therapy measures, and anti-inflammatory medications.

Through my interactions with these patients and listening to their struggles to find both a diagnosis and definitive treatment for their pain, my sense of what I can only call innate humanity and spirituality was reignited. It was truly a time of transformation for me as I listened to their stories, and heard how they'd been fighting an uphill battle with America's healthcare system. I learned how much they had suffered; in many cases losing friends, family and finances. These early patients taught me what institutions had not; about the severe pain this joint can cause, and the enormous inner strength it took to endure and still maintain hope. These patients were true pioneers and pilgrims on their journeys for pain relief.

A major breakthrough for me came as a result of a 2001 symposium I organized, inviting experts and clinicians in chiropractic, physical therapy, psychiatry, rheumatology and osteopathy to share their experiences with chronic pain in this joint. Among these clinicians, many had a very good understanding of the diagnosis and multiple approaches for conservative treatments. I realized it was primarily the *surgeons*, both orthopedic and neurosurgeons, who had not been trained about chronic pain in the sacroiliac joint and had little or no knowledge about its diagnosis or treatments, both non-surgical and surgical.

Historically, people showing significant symptoms, such as severe pain, for which there was no known cure, were ostracized and isolated from their communities. They may have been considered "crazy" or "possessed." In our own country, decades of over-crowded asylums attest to this. With the progression of modern medicine, many of these conditions have been treated or cured. However, even though we now have a standard way to diagnose the dysfunctional sacroiliac joint, the surgical system in America does not teach surgeons to look for this as a potential pain generator when conducting medical history and clinical exams on patients. Despite the fact that it has been established that the sacroiliac joint is either one of or *the* prime pain generator for 15-22% of all new low back pain patients **(ref 1,2,3)**, tens of thousands of people seen yearly by primary care doctors, orthopedic and neurosurgeons are unlikely to be checked for this condition. However, clinicians who aren't surgeons readily diagnose this condition and have a good success rate using manual treatments or injections.

This book is not about those whose pain is eliminated through conservative methods; it is about thousands of others for whom these measures have failed, received only temporary relief, chronically suffer and qualify for a surgical solution. Although several surgeries for fusion of this joint have appeared in medical literature over the last century, it continues to be ignored by medical schools, residency programs, orthopedic and neurosurgical spine fellowships, as well as major surgical educational societies. There are no questions on board exams by either the American Orthopedic or Neurosurgical Board of Examiners concerning surgery for the painful sacroiliac joint. While modern surgery is now curing pain caused by all the major joints in the body, such as hip, knee and spine, through fusion surgery or putting in new joints, the sacroiliac is still not being appropriately addressed by the surgical medical system or its educational and board examining societies. How can this be?

The answer to this question lies right at the heart of America's capitalistic healthcare system. It was the surgical device manufacturing industry that clearly recognized people did indeed suffer from chronic sacroiliac joint pain, that no standard for surgical treatment had emerged from the surgical educational societies, and an antiquated approach was used in trauma surgery to stabilize this joint. If they could create something similar to that approach, which pre-dated the Federal Drug Administration and thus eliminate oversight from that organization and costly pre-market approval, they could potentially make huge profits.

Throughout these pages I will explain how industry did manage to modernize a procedure for fusing the sacroiliac joint that pre-dated the FDA, and create a standard that has, over the past decade, become the one and only way for surgically treating chronic pain in this joint. I will discuss how over just a few years the number of these surgeries has escalated into the thousands; with one source even suggesting that possibly 50,000 of these fusions will be performed annually by the year 2020. Considering that the devices manufactured by industry and used in these surgeries average $10,000 each, the financial incentive is enormous.

Who is teaching surgeons how to perform these thousands of sacroiliac joint fusions each year since it is not the medical schools and surgical educational societies performing these duties? It is the surgical device industry that has taken over this crucial role and managed to become the sole driver for these surgeries. They not only create the instrumentation to be used in these procedures, they also educate surgeons on how to use them and "over-help" in the solicitation of patients. While maintaining significant forward momentum, they have also rendered the entire surgical educational system, which should be concerned with providing surgical solutions for chronic sacroiliac joint pain, totally impotent. They have accomplished this by offering significant financial gain to the very surgeons responsible for providing the highest level of non-biased and scientifically driven education and research for all aspects of chronic back pain. This has created an enormous conflict of interest for many of our surgical educational leaders. As for the patients, they get whatever industry is handing out, which currently comes with a "one procedure fits all attitude." Although this one type of surgery does have a 75% success rate, the following pages will offer much insight as to the negative aspects for patients who receive surgical healthcare using this model.

Twenty-six years have passed since I performed my first joint fusion for chronic sacroiliac pain, and I am now retired. Over the years, I have performed hundreds of these surgeries. From a personal perspective, this venture has consisted of cutting-edge surgical science, with its successes and failures along the way. But there has been an enormous spiritual component as well. I had been raised to consider all of humanity as being equal, and that whatever I did in order to help another should be done using my best efforts. This led me to create ways to surgically treat people suffering with chronic pain. This approach took me frequently into uncharted areas of surgical methods and techniques that, being untested, relied on sensible logic and very trusting patients. My early surgical ideas took me into parts of the body about which I had not been fully trained by my educators for these purposes. Surgeries, by their very nature, can be full of surprises, and in order to navigate them successfully requires some "faith" and "commitment" on the part of the surgeon, the patient, and the whole surgical team. Whenever I felt a situation in the O.R. was becoming precarious, the team would always come together as a unified spirit; wanting the absolute best outcome for each patient. This was true whether the declared faiths in the room were Muslim, Christian, Judaism, or any other. My experiences taught me that treating people with chronic pain involves many very dedicated and caring individuals working together for the common good.

I have written this book because this diagnosis continues to be largely ignored by the medical community as a common reason for low back pain. I could not have accomplished it without the help and shared experiences of several colleagues, to whom I am eternally grateful. My goal is to inform the general public, give them tools to seek further information, ask the right questions to better understand the source of their chronic pain, and give them hope that it might be resolved.

You will meet some of my patients throughout this book. Their names have been changed, but it is the substance of their stories that is important for many readers who have similar experiences.

For those wanting a "fast track" through this book, reading the **"Being Your Own Advocate"** sections at the end of each chapter, along with the chapters titled **"The Sacroiliac Playbook"**, and **"How To Be Your Own Advocate"** will provide an overview, tools and a helpful start in the search for pain resolution.

Bruce E Dall, MD

2017

Disclaimer: The contents of this book are considered to be for general educational purposes only and are in no way meant to be construed as medical treatment. The author claims no responsibility for any adverse outcomes that might result from anyone following the advice given in this book. Before deciding to commit to any form of treatment, conservative or surgical, individuals should consult with their doctor.

Introduction

A classic case of the chronic dysfunctional sacroiliac joint.

Lucy had just made an agonizing decision. She could no longer have sex with her husband due to increasing pain that was now too great to bear. It had started as an unpleasant physical annoyance but had become so severe it now caused her overwhelming anxiety in both the anticipation, and the unbearable pain during what had now become a frightening ordeal. She knew what was causing the pain; both her physical therapist and pain doctor had explained that it was her left sacroiliac joint. Lucy didn't fully understand what this joint was, but she knew that everyone has two, and they were the two large joints holding the spine to the pelvis, the boney cradle in which Lucy's babies, years ago, had developed and passed through during childbirth **(Fig 1)**.

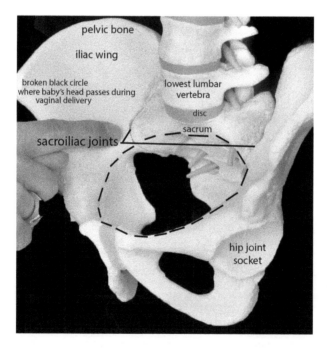

Fig 1. Looking inside the pelvic bone from the front, the

anterior portions of the sacroiliac joints are seen as part of the pelvic ring (broken lines) that a baby's head must pass through during birth. The sacroiliac joints at this point spread open to allow this circle to become temporarily larger. Although both men and women suffer from pain due to the sacroiliac, giving birth is a common origin of this condition in females.

Lucy had been receiving periodic injections, but they gave her only temporary relief. The rest of the time her pain was constant. Certain activities, like making love, made it much worse. Standing, sitting and even lying on her left side caused unrelenting pain. After four years of this, Lucy was not only suffering physically, but emotionally. Because her intense pain limited her abilities and energy, she had lost her job, many of her friends, and now her marriage was on the line. She was desperate and had little hope that anything would change.

I had heard Lucy's story, and others like it, from hundreds of women and men over the past three decades, and it is still being played out today by thousands more across the country. All suffer from a condition called a "dysfunctional sacroiliac joint." As a result, people like Lucy, for whom traditional treatments have failed, are forced to live with significant chronic pain. Another group of patients, possibly larger, consists of people with disabling chronic low back pain, which has not been diagnosed. These men and women may have had one or more unsuccessful back surgeries, including fusions. For them, it is even more depressing, having to suffer with this painful condition because the medical system is not equipped to diagnose or manage it. In my experience, and that of many other spine surgeons, the sacroiliac joint has turned out to be the cause of this pain in many of these misunderstood and frequently misdiagnosed individuals.

Chapter 1

Joan, How It All Began

*How a remarkable patient inspired me to create a surgical
solution during "the Golden Age of Medicine".*

When I first saw Joan entering my clinic from across the waiting
room, my initial instinct was pure fear. As she drew closer, that
feeling became mixed with uncertainty and compassion. It was
interesting that throughout medical school, and in all my training
since, there had been no preparation for dealing with any of these
emotions. Fear was never to be discussed or outwardly shown.
Expressing fear was akin to peeing your pants in public, as that is
how both teachers and peers would view you. Uncertainty was not
an option; doctors were trained, even if not directly, to develop and
carry an air of certainty regardless of the situation. The concept of
compassion rarely came up. There were a few of my mentors who
did show what I would call compassion to patients, but in general I
was taught that doctors were to be objective, and not become
attached, as it might compromise their ability to do the best job
possible. I continue to feel that many doctors who exhibit true
compassion either possess it naturally or developed it from parents
or other role models. It would be a good thing if medical schools
had a course on how to demonstrate compassion to patients and
that it is okay to do so.

As I stood at the clinic's elbow-height counter, signing orders for a
patient I had just seen, Joan was being rolled toward me in a
wheelchair, accompanied by her three daughters. The intense look
on each of their faces conveyed not only apprehension, but also a
very clear message that said, "You better help our mom, or else!". I
was five years into my career as an orthopedic surgeon, but already
familiar with the fierce determination of sons or daughters who
accompanied a sick parent. I willed myself to appear in control,
demonstrate assurance, and convey a caring attitude. Of course, I
did sincerely care a great deal, but at this point in my practice I was
still questioning whether I had what it took to handle these
situations professionally, and get the respect I so badly wanted from
my colleagues. As I watched Joan and her family approach, despite
my best efforts to appear confident, I couldn't dispel the feeling of
dread that was welling up inside. At that moment, and on many

occasions to come, I wholeheartedly wished I had learned coping skills to deal with these types of feelings; not only as a doctor, but even as a child and adolescent. I had grown up in an immigrant neighborhood and attended a high school where only 29% of graduates went on to college. My paternal grandparents emigrated from Denmark at the dawn of the twentieth century and brought with them their state religion of Lutheranism. Growing up in this strict religious environment did not allow for the expression or understanding of emotions. The best way for a child to survive was to keep a closed lip and just follow the rules.

As a boy, I seemed to be in fights constantly, since, in our Midwest neighborhood, Lutherans and Catholics were not friends. (I actually did become Catholic, later in life, after meeting my wife), but it was from these early experiences I learned that showing any emotion was a form of weakness. Despite this, I was very lucky to find some wonderful role models who helped me navigate my way through high school and into college. It was my student council sponsor who, for some unknown reason, made it her goal that I should go to college. While still an undergraduate, it was my father-in-law-to-be who convinced me I had what it took to direct my energies toward medical school. Since my parents and older siblings had not continued their education beyond high school, it represented a small miracle that I managed to end up in college and a very large miracle that medical school came next. Since I had received so much love and support from these individuals and so many more afterwards, I was resolved to pursue a profession in which I could help people. Little did I know that dealing with my emotions would be something I would only start to master after commencing my career at the age of thirty-three. I also did not realize at the time I treated Joan, that she would prove to be not only one of my biggest challenges, both medically and emotionally, but that she would, in many ways, define how I would go on to think about patients and medicine.

As we moved into the exam room, with all three of Joan's daughters talking at once, I managed to gather that Joan had been suffering for several years. Her pain had now progressed to the point where she could no longer walk. She had severe rheumatoid arthritis, and at 74, was nearly overcome by it. Her future, and even her life, were being threatened. Joan's most severe pain was in her right buttock, radiating from the back of her leg down through her foot. She sat perched on her left buttock while simultaneously pushing down on the right armrest. She had a look of despair, but still, her eyes seemed to hold a glimmer of hope. From her daughters, I learned this arthritic condition had caused Joan's right sacroiliac joint to disconnect, which was proven by a CT scan, showing the joint was separated by almost 1/2 an inch. Another test, a bone scan, revealed intense abnormal activity in this joint, which indicated there was tremendous potential for pain. The sacroiliac is a joint that literally holds together the entire spine and pelvis. It is the core of the body's need for ultimate stability in performing even the most menial of activities. The sacrum is the lowest bone in the spine and is shaped like a shield or triangle. With the spine attached at the top and shortest part of this triangle, the pelvis is attached to each of its two long sides. These connections are the sacroiliac joints **(Fig. 1)**. A cross section of a painful sacroiliac joint is shown below **(Fig.2)**

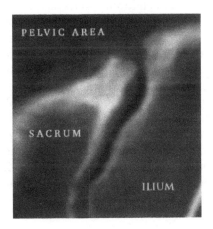

Fig 2. A CT scan showing a cross sectional view of an arthritic sacroiliac joint. The ilium in this scan is the same as the iliac wing in Fig 1. The black in the joint is nitrogen gas, which can be part of the picture of arthritis. The increased white areas are increased bone density to handle the additional stresses of a degenerating joint.

In 1991, when this story took place, my knowledge of the sacroiliac was limited. I understood where the joints were located, that they should, if healthy, be stable and show minimal or no movement. They weren't typically a significant source for pain, unless, for example, in a pregnant woman near term or someone who had been through a physical trauma such as a car accident or fall, which could rip them apart. Now I was faced with a patient whose very unstable and painful sacroiliac was causing profound disability, although she was neither young, pregnant, and had not had a major traumatic event. I was about to learn very quickly that medical and surgical science had not yet caught up on effective treatments for this woman's problem.

The year 1991 represents a time when surgical treatment for spinal conditions was going through a major transition, similar to the advent of surgical instrumentation in the 1950s. In 1953, Dr. Paul Harrington at Baylor College of Medicine in Texas developed the "Harrington Rod," to be used in children and teens for the diagnosis of scoliosis or curvature of the spine. This device proved so successful that its same instrumentation was utilized to realign and stabilize fractured or broken spines in the 1980s. By the time Joan sought my help, the use of screws and plates to stabilize the spine was just beginning. We had learned from the previous breakthroughs that if segments of the spine, either for scoliosis or trauma, were stabilized, then had ground-up pelvic bone placed along the length of the hardware, that a fusion, or a biological weld would occur. This would then hold the spine in that position hopefully forever. The screws and plates in these early spine surgeries were the same as those employed to bind the fractured bones of arms or legs to allow natural healing.

Many professionals in the surgical business consider this time to have been the "Golden Age of Medicine." For Joan, it meant that a surgeon was not only allowed to come up with his or her own solutions, but was even encouraged to do so by colleagues, hospitals, and informed patients. Unfortunately, in order to move the science of surgical medicine along, patients often became guinea pigs. Depending on the circumstances and the surgeon, these trial and error efforts could result in either desirable or undesirable outcomes.

As I continued to listen to Joan, examine her, and review all her scans, it began to sink in just how hopeless her situation seemed. I learned that she had been to the Mayo Clinic and to University of Michigan Hospital. Along the way, she had seen several orthopedic surgeons, and the message she received repeatedly was, yes, her sacroiliac joint was separated, and was complicated by her rheumatoid arthritis, but no surgery could help her. She was warned that should surgery be attempted, it would more than likely fail and her life would be at extreme risk. Joan had been referred to me by an acquaintance I had treated successfully for a more run-of-the-mill spine surgery. She told me she truly believed I was her last hope. If I could not help her, she felt her only choice was to end her life, as she could no longer endure the pain. She was the most desperate person I had met at this point in my career.

Prior to Joan, I had limited experience in surgically treating the sacroiliac joint, especially in an elderly woman with rheumatoid arthritis. Although I was part of a large surgical practice, I knew my partners had no more experience than I did. But I was well trained, had published papers on problems near this joint, and my goal at this early stage in my profession was to save the world! There was not much in my personal arsenal beyond a deep determination not to abandon this woman, and to do everything I possibly could to help alleviate her suffering. Something inside me was saying, "stay the course, it will be all right." In the years following, after I had seen many patients like Joan, some in even worse shape, those words continued to come back to me like a private mantra. My desire to help Joan occurred during a time when doing whatever you could come up with was still considered something like the "Good Samaritan Law", (which provides basic legal protection for one who assists a person who is injured or in danger) even if the end result was not always favorable. I did not know then that a decade later, restrictions regarding this type of "creative license" would no longer be allowed. What I learned from treating Joan would prove to be invaluable for many future patients as time moved forward.

So, I asked myself, was it faith that was moving me on or my unchecked youthful ego? That question could be posed to many a man or woman throughout history as they ventured into the unknown to pursue their passion for a good cause. I told Joan I would have to do some research, but if I could create a surgical approach that made sense, I would offer it to her. She in turn said she would pray for me, and left the office flanked by her daughters, to await my call.

As I pondered where to go from here, (and considered praying myself), I thought about what I actually knew concerning surgery for this joint. After all, it had certainly been operated on before; for decades there had existed a method for stabilizing the sacroiliac when it had been subjected to trauma. Typically, this involved making a large incision across the buttock, dissecting its muscles off the pelvis and inserting two long bone screws across the sacroiliac joint, from the pelvic bone, across the sacroiliac joint and into the sacral bone. This served to realign and hold the joint in place while the surrounding ligaments healed and provided internal stabilization. This procedure relieved pain permanently in about half of these patients, but the remaining 50% went on to suffer chronic disabling pain.

Because of this, and the fact that with rheumatoid arthritis, such as Joan's, comes osteoporosis, or weak, fragile bones, screws put in this way would likely not hold well. This is why Joan, until now, had not been considered a viable candidate for surgery. I agreed that this catchall surgery was not a good option. If these screws were put in they would loosen and pull out, leaving her in even worse condition. It happened that other research I had been conducting on a different approach to pelvic problems, led me to come up with a surgical alternative (albeit very cautiously and possibly with some divine intervention). that I believed had a chance of working. It had never been done before, but by utilizing all the resources I was able to muster from concepts of the "old masters," along with adapting newer techniques, which had proven successful for traditional spinal problems, I believed we now had a chance.

The essence of this surgery revolved around concepts I had published in 1994 on how to surgically approach the pelvic bone through one straight incision directly on the back and gently separating layers of muscles and fascia without cutting through them. From there the actual sacroiliac joint could be directly approached and visualized. This would also allow more modern screws and plates to be inserted more securely at angles different from the "two screws from the lateral side approach." It would provide for better bone grafting and stabilization in someone with decreased bone density. It would also allow for a better surgical closure and faster rehabilitation after surgery.

Joan and her daughters returned to my office, where I explained my idea as carefully and precisely as I could. I let them know in no uncertain terms that this type of procedure had never been performed, and had a definite chance of failing, yet, if it did work, it could decrease her pain and increase her function. Joan's response was, "I trust you, let's get on with it!"

As an adolescent, the only doctor I knew was Dr. A.C. Anderson. Remembering him brought back the god-like images I had conjured up as a youngster. He had been our family doctor for years and my mother gave him full credit for saving her on more than one occasion. Everything he said was absolutely true and everything he did was for the absolute good. When I was 15 months old I drank half a glass of ammonia my mother had placed in the oven to air it out. Dr. Anderson sat in my bedroom through most of that night, ready to intubate me if necessary. Later, he removed my tonsils, then my appendix. Although we often sat in his waiting room for hours before being seen, we had nothing but gratitude for this man, in whom we had unwavering trust and respect. It suddenly struck me that Joan was regarding me now in the same way my mother and I had looked at our doctor, who, to us, was a real-life hero. Joan was turning herself over to me, for better or worse. She had abiding faith that I would proceed with only her best interest at heart. I wished then I could be more like Dr. Anderson; bold, courageous, unflinching and seemingly able to bear the weight of the world on his shoulders. Instead, I felt as though a huge boulder was weighing me down, and I was not entirely confident I could carry it.

Seven days later, with all the i's dotted and all the t's crossed, we headed for the operating room. I remember nothing else about that day except every single second of Joan's entire surgery. My focus was so intense that everything taking place was forever branded into my brain. I was very lucky to have the chief resident of orthopedics, Joe Perra, as my assistant. He had just been accepted into one of the country's premier orthopedic spine fellowships, and this procedure had piqued his interest. His mind was sharp, and I knew he would be one of the best people to have by my side as I worked through this new technique. Joe would later go on to become one of a select few; an internationally renowned and respected spine surgeon. He and I would talk two and a half decades later, recount Joan's surgery together, and he would share the experience with his orthopedic residents and spine fellows.

Joan was now asleep, facedown on the table, and her back had been prepped and draped. I began by making a long, straight incision in the middle of her back from her waist to her tailbone. Thanks to the research I had done, I was able to expose her right posterior pelvic bone, with very little blood loss and no tissue disruption, and after cutting the deepest muscles over the lower spine in half and reflecting them out of the way, I was able to view the entire back of the sacrum's and pelvis's right side. A portion of the pelvic bone was removed with an instrument called a "rongeur", which looks much like the mouth of a Tyrannosaurus Rex on the end of a large pair of pliers. Removing this bone allowed us to see deep into the sacroiliac joint, and the same bone would be used as bone graft material for the fusion. We were working in a very vascular part of the body; so keeping the bleeding controlled was paramount. I was thankful that we had a "cautery," a pen-like device that generates an electric current through its tip and literally fries the blood vessels closed. Because the pelvic bone is very porous, the bite taken out of it by the "T Rex" would cause blood to ooze from the bone. To stem the hemorrhage, we had pushed bone wax into the tiny holes. Blood was already hanging on an IV pole should we need it, but Joan remained stable. The sacroiliac joint was now visible! This was the first time I had seen it in a live patient, something I later discovered I shared with only a few orthopedic surgeons in America at that time, and perhaps the world. This joint, which should have been rigidly stable, showing no movement, was sprung open about 1/2 an inch. The bones of the sacrum and pelvis, which should join to make this joint, looked nearly disconnected. My consternation increased as I realized that any screws or other instrumentation I inserted would have to hold firmly in these two bones in order to fixate the sacroiliac joint between them. Using the "T. Rex" device, the arthritic inside of the joint was cleaned out, or "debrided" and grafting material from the pelvic bone removed earlier was packed into it. Eventually, it would turn to solid bone and heal the pelvis to the sacrum, just as a fracture heals, thus completely stabilizing it. The next challenge was deciding which hardware to choose. The spinal screws and rods, which would become standard in the ensuing five years, did not yet exist. The Harrington Rod for scoliosis would not work for this operation. Our best option was the same fixation used to plate the long bone of the thigh, or "femur," after a fracture. The idea was to take this plate, which was stainless steel with holes in it, and insert large 6.5mm screws at each end and attach pelvis to sacrum, crossing the joint, which I had previously filled with bone graft.

It was here we ran into a big snag. The shortest plate we had was six inches long, twice the length we needed. The plates were 3/8 of an inch thick, solid steel, and impossible for us to cut. Our only option was to rush the plate down to the hospital's engineering department, have it cut to our specifications, and sent back immediately, where it would be resterilized and inserted.

I had never before stopped for an undetermined amount of time during a surgery, and I knew the longer it took, the more blood Joan would lose, putting her at increased risk. The plate was returned forty minutes later, although the wait had seemed like hours. Working as fast as possible, we placed it across the joint and inserted the two screws into what appeared to be good bone. As each was tightened, we were enormously relieved to see they were holding firmly and would not strip out. With the hardware in place, I performed the "Kube Shake Test." Dr. Kube had been a teacher in my residency and following a procedure like this, he would grab whatever hardware had been implanted into bone with heavy pliers and forcefully attempt to pull it out. I held my breath as I timidly grasped the plate, and then with greater strength, tried to pull on it. Nothing budged, and with a tremendous sigh, Joe and I began reconstructing layers of muscle, fascia and skin to close the incision.

Nine years after several more successful surgeries on patients with chronic sacroiliac pain, I heard that Joan had passed away. She had gone to the emergency room for a heart condition unrelated to her surgery, and while in the E.R., an X-Ray of her abdomen had been taken which also happened to include her pelvis. It showed the plate and screws I had put in place were still holding firmly, not having moved. **(Fig 3).**

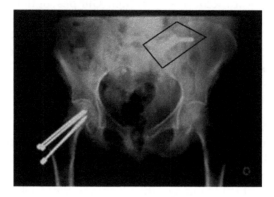

**Fig 3. Joan's X-Ray nine years following surgery. The
black enclosed area shows the plate and screws used to
fuse the sacroiliac joint together, which had not shifted or
become loose.**

Joan's family shared with me that because of her arthritis; she had
still used a walker right up until a week before she died. However,
she had not suffered from back pain since her surgery. Two years
later I published Joan's case in the *Journal of Orthopedics and
Techniques.*

Joan had lived a remarkable life. She embodied the spirit of a
pioneer woman who stood strong against all odds, and embraced
her faith, which gave her the belief that all would work out, as it
should.

There were many lessons to be learned from Joan, but I would not
fully appreciate them until I was older and more experienced. At
the time, I freely admit my ego was soaring, making it hard to be
spiritually centered and get beyond the thrill that my own invention
had been a complete success! But trying times were yet to come,
and when they did, I was able to survive by relying on the faith
shown to me by Joan and other exceptional people in my life.

Being Your Own Advocate
Lessons from Joan

1 Living with chronic pain can lead someone to thoughts of ending his or her life rather than continuing to endure it. It is important to keep searching for a cure as the medical system is rapidly changing. This is a time in your life when turning to whatever it is that you have faith in might benefit you in the long run.

2 Utilize all the advocates you can to be your voice if you are unable to be your own.

3 Just because major medical centers do not fully grasp your diagnosis when it comes to sacroiliac joint pain doesn't mean the answer is not out there, somewhere.

4 It is crucial that you find a surgeon you trust completely to treat your pain and fully turn over control to that person.

5 If surgery removes your pain, it is essential to get on with your life and live it to the fullest.

Chapter 2
My Sacroiliac Joint Education

An overview of the early concepts of sacroiliac joint pain and its treatment, and

how it became my mission to help those afflicted with this condition.

The sacroiliac joint is still something of an enigma. Despite the fact that every person on earth has two of them, most would be hard-pressed to locate them. The words "sacro-iliac" are used in phrases like, "I got a pain in my sacroiliac," and have shown up in song lyrics by artists ranging from Sinatra to Chubby Checker to 10cc's "C'mon Mac, do the sacroiliac." The general take on the word seems to be that it has something to do with the back and back pain, the buttock, movement, functions and feelings. The word is used in ways that imply an unknown "something" that is intrinsically part of our back, but has no specific definition. It has been defined anatomically since the days of Greek physician Hippocrates, but otherwise has not been clearly understood like the hip, knee or ankle. Many medical practitioners still have no unified understanding of its purpose, how much it moves, how it causes pain or how it relates to the surrounding anatomy.

The word "fusion" in relation to surgery on the sacroiliac joint simply means to create a bridge of bone through the joint, thus locking the bone on one side to the bone on the other so no movement is possible. The first documented fusion was performed in 1878 by Viennese Professor Albert Early, who was treating a patient's painful arthritic knee. He opened the knee joint, removed the knee cap (patella), scraped cartilage from the joint ends of the leg bones (femur and tibia), positioned the knee cap between them, then placed the whole leg in a long plaster cast for nine months. When the cast was removed, the entire leg was solid from hip to ankle. Although the patient could no longer bend his knee, he was free from pain and able to return to full labor. This was one of the beginnings of surgically fusing a joint together in order to relieve the chronic pain of severe arthritis.

Dr. Smith-Peterson, an orthopedic surgeon who was born in

Norway, studied at Harvard and practiced in Boston, used this
concept to perform a series of sacroiliac joint fusions in the 1920s.
His procedure was, and still is, considered a horrific one, both to
perform and to endure **(ref 4)**. The incision was about a foot long,
arching over the posterior pelvic bone, followed by a dissection of
the buttock muscles (gluteus maximus, medius and minimus,) off
the outside of the pelvic wall (iliac crest). It was in the very lowest
part of this bloody dissection that this bone overlaid the sacroiliac
joint. A large triangular piece of the iliac crest was removed with
chisels and the joint underneath was scraped free of cartilage. The
iliac bone triangle was turned and its boney side was impacted into
the hole. After this extremely aggressive approach and bone work,
the next enormous task was to stop all bleeding and close the wound
layer by layer, using a barbaric suturing technique. A plaster cast
was then applied, reaching from the nipple line to to the ankle on
the fusion side, and the hip joint on the other. The patient was bed-
ridden and required round-the-clock assistance for the next nine
months. Although Dr. Smith-Peterson reported a very satisfactory
success rate, he failed to mention any of the complications and
morbidities that were part of his patients' experience.

The surgical/medical society at that time in history had not
progressed far in terms of treatment for the ubiquitous malady of
low back pain. As the only moveable joint in the pelvis, the
sacroiliac was blamed not only for most pain of the lower back, but
for almost every case of "sciatica" or radiating leg pain. This was in
large part due to the early publications by Dr. Smith-Peterson. It
was generally believed that this pain was caused by traumatic
arthritis and tuberculosis, as other explanations for pain in this
joint had yet to be discovered. All of this was occurring before the
"herniated lumbar disk," now considered the source of the majority
of low back and leg pain, was even known to be a pathological
entity.

There was a positive side here for patients; being diagnosed with
sacroiliac joint arthritis or disease for one's persistent and often-
disabling back and leg pain, was a blessing for many sufferers. Prior
to this, they were frequently admitted to psychiatric hospitals or
asylums since their symptoms had no identifiable medical origin,
and it was deemed to be "all in their heads." At least those who
received this more specific diagnosis were no longer ostracized. Not
everyone who received this pronouncement, however, was able to

have surgery, because only a few orthopedic surgeons had knowledge about this joint and were capable of performing such operations. In addition, most hospitals were unable to handle these types of major bloodletting procedures. For those who did undergo surgery, resulting complications and failures were seldom reported, so how these patients fared as a group remains something of a mystery. The claim was that approximately 75% improved, but beyond that very little was divulged. Despite terse reporting on results, these early pioneers in surgery did establish that the sacroiliac joint could cause pain, provided an extensive review of its anatomical location, and demonstrated that fusing this joint might provide relief. But in the year 1934, this all became moot.

The third decade of the twentieth century is when surgical medicine for low back and leg pain took a giant step out of the dark ages. Massachusetts General Hospital surgeons Mixter and Barr operated on a patient's back after finding a questionable tumor within the spinal canal, by using a new diagnostic tool called the "myelogram". The myelogram involved being stuck with a very large bore needle, deep into the spine through the thin sac (dura) containing spinal fluid. This was followed by something like the equivalent of today's 10W30 motor oil injected into the spinal fluid; the heavy oil would appear as a black mass on what were then primitive X-Rays, and could be monitored as it flowed through the spinal canal. To allow the oil to gravitate from the low back to the head, while avoiding the brain (which would have been catastrophic), the patient had to be positioned practically on their head. If the oil stopped moving, something was obstructing the spinal canal. The obstruction could not be identified until the surgeon actually went in and explored the area. Mixter and Barr fully expected to discover a tumor in the spinal canal, putting pressure on all the nerves but instead, after examining the tissue they surgically removed from their patient under a microscope, they found the tissue consistent with a lumbar disc. The lumbar disc is the tissue separating each of the vertebral bones throughout the entire spine. What they learned was the soft center of this hockey-puck shaped disc could explode from its walls and into the spinal canal, exerting pressure on the spinal nerves. Once they removed the obstruction, the patient improved dramatically. Subsequently, they published an account of their extruded disc removal and shortly thereafter, most all back and leg pain was widely attributed, without much exception, to the herniated disc. Simultaneously, the former belief about the sacroiliac joint's ability to cause back and leg pain fell into oblivion.

It would be over 50 years before the next study on surgery for this joint would appear in medical literature.

Medical professionals of the mid-twentieth century now had a new and definitive diagnosis for all low back and leg pain (rheumatic and sciatica), which they embraced as gospel and looked no further into the sacroiliac joint as a major pain source. If a patient with pain in these areas had a negative myelogram, showing no spinal canal obstruction, it meant there was no legitimate explanation for their suffering, and they often ended up labeled as a "crock", or in today's terms, a hypochondriac or even "nutcase." Many lived out their lives in constant pain and some were even institutionalized.

We now know many of these people were suffering from chronically painful sacroiliac joints. It's ironic that these same patients, who would have been correctly diagnosed and treated in the 20s, half a century later might as well have been living in the Middle Ages; thought to be conjuring with spirits and demons. Since I know of at least two suicides in the past decade by individuals diagnosed with sacroiliac joint pain who were unable to receive an adequate diagnosis or treatment, my guess is that the number of those who ended their own lives between the 1940s and 1980s was probably much higher.

I began my medical education in South Omaha where I had grown up, at the University of Nebraska Medical Center, not far from the region's major employer and world's largest stockyard. How I ended up a medical student, considering my background as the grandson of a laboring immigrant family, is one of many miracles in my life. It was 1978, shortly before the sacroiliac joint was to emerge from fifty years of "hibernation," when, as a third year med student, I encountered my first so-called "crock" patient while on clinical rounds with the chief medical resident and her entourage of residents.

Being a medical student in that environment at that time was very daunting and sometimes humiliating. If they could make you cry, it would, as "Dirty Harry" later famously said, "make their day." I was expected to do an entire consultation on a patient new to this group, then present every detail, no matter how minor, that I could uncover. Afterward, my superiors would grill me until I was at least "well done." Bill, one of my patients at that time, was a middle-aged man who'd been suffering low back pain for at least four years. The onset of his pain began after a car accident he had been in while intoxicated. The car he was driving left the road and hit a telephone pole head-on. He remembered slamming his right foot on the brake and bracing for impact. After sobering up and not having any broken bones the hospital released him. Subsequently, he suffered from continuous severe low back pain. Although he had seen a few doctors in the past few years, no accurate diagnosis was made and no treatment recommended. The pain was in his right lower back and radiated down his right leg. He had now reached the point where he had difficulty walking and could not hold a job. Clinically, Bill's pain was identified as being over his right buttock and down the back of his thigh to the knee. All his nerves were working; he had no muscle weakness and could feel everything. The key reflexes in his knees and ankles were normal. He also had normal back X-Rays and lumbar myelogram. Although I didn't have much to go on, I presented this to my expert panel of judges. Before I even finished, Sarah, the chief resident proclaimed, "Oh, he's just a crock - let's move on to the next patient." There wasn't any inkling in her tone that she was talking about an actual human being.

I was not used to anyone being treated like this. Even though I pretty much fought my way through growing up in South Omaha, at least you looked eye-to-eye at whoever was about to thrust their knuckles in your face, and you considered each other and everyone else in the neighborhood equals. Dismissing someone out-of-hand was foreign to me. I never forgot that encounter. I also never thought at the time I would be spending the bulk of my future career as an orthopedic spine surgeon trying to diagnose patients like Bill. Neither did I understand that Bill's mechanism of injury, braking with a right straight leg at the time of a front-end impact, would come to be recognized as a classic way to severely injure the sacroiliac joint on that side, or that I would publish such accounts in future literature. Making a reasonable diagnosis for a patient having back and leg pain was not considered possible in the 1970s without a positive myelogram. This test had become the absolute objective evidence necessary for creation of such symptoms. If you, as a doctor, were to suggest some other cause for this pain, such as the sacroiliac joint, you were considered as "crazy" as the patient.

What I did learn in my nine years of surgical education was that the sacroiliac joint caused pain in near-term pregnant women, secondary to hormonal changes, resulting in the ligaments holding the two joints together becoming more elastic. This was in preparation for the baby's head to exit the pelvis by allowing the pelvic bones to spread apart. In roughly three to five percent of these women, the result was a large dose of low back and leg pain. In most cases this intense pain would abate in the weeks following delivery, as hormones reversed and ligaments tightened back up. If the pain did not go away and if there was no other explanation, these women fell into the "crock" or "head case" designation. Other accepted causes for persistent sacroiliac joint pain were a healed fracture or infection. The residual of both could be viewed on an X-Ray, so patients were given validation for their pain. Interestingly, we would later learn that the X-Ray findings of the sacroiliac joint, except in cases of trauma, infection or tumor, would have zero correlation with chronic sacroiliac dysfunctional pain.

At that time, there were really only two types of surgeries being done on the sacroiliac joint, if a surgeon was astute enough to make the diagnosis. I was not yet one of them. The first employed the Smith-Peterson technique, now sixty to seventy years old and still regarded as barbaric. The other, as a result of bone screws invented in the 1940s, was used when acute trauma ripped the joint apart, separating the pelvis from the sacrum. This surgery consisted of placing two big bone screws through the pelvic bone, across the sacroiliac joint, and into the sacral bone. Using X-Rays intra-operatively and keeping the screws within anatomical boundaries made this surgery possible. This did hold the joint together in an anatomical position, but no effort was made to fuse the joint to make it solid. Fifty percent of these patients went on to endure chronic and often disabling low back, many with associated leg pain. No further treatment was available surgically except to remove the screws, on the theory they may be causing the pain, but this rarely helped.

By the 1980s and with the invention of the CT scan, with the exception of tumors, fractures and infections we now had three accepted diagnoses for pain in the low back and legs; the herniated lumbar disc, spinal stenosis (blockage of the spinal canal from arthritis pressing on nerves), and the still not well-understood sacroiliac joint. Over the next thirty years, the herniated disc and spinal stenosis continued to take center stage as primary causes for this sort of pain, leaving the sacroiliac joint recognized as a real entity, but basically ignored as an essential cause of this type of malady. There were no requirements for an orthopedic spine surgeon or neurosurgeon to know anything about this joint as a chronic pain generator. Surgeons were not obliged to understand the anatomy surrounding this joint, how to diagnose it as a pain generator, or how to surgically treat it, other than with a brutal seventy-year-old procedure or a dated and most often-ineffective trauma technique. If a patient with this problem went to an orthopedic surgeon's office, and we now know tens of thousands did, they were likely to be promptly dismissed. When I met Joan, my first sacroiliac joint patient, I realized from that point on that how to diagnose and treat someone with severe chronic pain stemming from the sacroiliac joint was going to be entirely up to me.

Being Your Own Advocate
Lessons from my early Surgical Education

1 Surgeries to fuse the sacroiliac joint for chronic low back pain have been performed successfully for nearly a century.

2 It is important to obtain an accurate diagnosis for your chronic low back pain.

3 Since orthopedic and neurosurgical spine surgeons receive no formal training on how to diagnose and treat, either conservatively or surgically, the chronically painful sacroiliac joint, you must seek out a surgeon with an open mind and an active interest in this joint.

Chapter 3
Beware the Light-Haired, Fair-Skinned Woman
The role genetics can play in sacroiliac joint pain.

Laurie was the first patient who actually made a 500-mile trek across a time zone to see me. I had now been operating on the painful sacroiliac joint for over ten years and had published one paper on the subject. It was 2002. I was now receiving referrals from doctors, surgeons and physical therapists throughout my community, as I had given talks locally and had personally spoken to many of these practitioners about my beliefs. In retrospect, I now see that I was living in a very small and well-circumscribed world in terms of patients and referral sources, and I felt comfortable in this environment. When Laurie first walked into my office, I had no way of knowing that much, if not the entire sacroiliac world I had been working to learn about for several years, was about to change dramatically.

Laurie's story initially surprised me, but as the years passed it would become a familiar one, being relayed by people literally all over the globe. Laurie was in her late thirties and had three small children. Her pain had begun with the birth of her first child, a son, delivered vaginally with a large head and weighing in at nearly ten pounds. Her description of how this little dude tore her apart on his way out, and how much surgical repair she needed, made me (not for the first time) thankful that as a man I would never have to endure this ordeal.

The culprit behind Laurie's ongoing pain turned out to be her genetic profile. She was a thin, light-haired, freckled woman of Northern European descent. It so happens that many women, and some men, who satisfy these same criteria share a genetic "error" in their collagen metabolism. Collagen is the tissue that holds us together and consists of bone, ligaments (which hold the joints together) and several of the body's structures including the inner lining of blood vessels, the sclera (white part of the eye), and many others. This inborn anomaly, due to a small genetic change in DNA, produces less than normal amounts of collagen. Anyone who fits this profile and whose joints are "hypermobile" (loose joints that can move beyond the normal range of motion), stands a chance of falling into this category **(Fig 4)**.

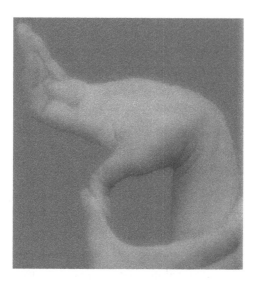

Fig 4. This photo shows both a hypermobile wrist and thumb. These extremes of joint motion can be associated with loose or lax ligaments. These structures are made of collagen fibrils which can have genetic inborn errors allowing for excessive stretching and more joint motion. When joint mobility like this is present, the ligaments holding the sacroiliac joints together could be affected as well and could result in painful conditions.

One of my first publications as an orthopedic surgeon was on this very subject, involving data from women I had seen in my clinical practice who had hypermobility in their hands, which positively correlated with osteopenia (less bone density) **(Ref 5)**. The problem with this type of genetic make-up is that if the ligaments and joint capsule for the sacroiliac joints lack the full complement of collagen fibrils for strength and resilience and when vigorously stretched (as in childbirth), these supporting ligaments can be injured. The ligaments and capsule are then not able to provide adequate support and stability for the SIJ from that point on, and can elicit varying degrees of chronic pain. OB and GYN doctors have recognized this injury for decades and many articles have appeared over the decades in their respective journals discussing the pain it can cause a young mother. Orthopedic surgeons as far back as the 1950s understood this problem often arose in young girls with painful loose shoulders and ankles. They knew when they performed a ligament repair to tighten one of these joints, there would be temporary relief, but within a short time they would simply stretch out again and the same chronic pain would return. Although surgeons of that era had no clue, and many still don't, that there might be a genetic basis for this, they had seen it happen often enough that a red flag went up whenever a fair, light-haired hypermobile female appeared in their office. My orthopedic residency chairman, Dr. Curtis Hanson, used to tell us to "beware the redhead" for these very reasons.

Laurie, of course, had no idea that she was unique in this way, nor do most others who share her condition. As she continued to relate her story, it was obvious to me that no one from whom she had sought help comprehended it either. Having lived for so long with constant and incapacitating pain, she made the courageous decision to undertake the long trip to my Kalamazoo office.

Laurie had low back pain that radiated down the back of her leg. Other people she knew with similar problems had sought and received relief. Her journey started with her family doctor, who ordered an MRI of her low back or lumbar spine. It was entirely normal. He put her on anti-inflammatory medication and sent her to physical therapy. The medication did not really help so she stopped taking it. It was her physical therapist who began to shed some light on what might be causing Laurie's pain.

Although surgeons in the modern era know next to nothing about chronic pain in the sacroiliac joint, physical therapists have been all over it for years. What they do best is diagnosing this joint as a pain generator in the appropriate patient. Although proper diagnosis is a very good first step, when it comes to treating it and ultimately removing the pain, especially in someone like Laurie, many times a P.T. can fall short. There is a logical explanation for this in terms of anatomy. The way physical therapy works for any chronic joint pain in the body is to strengthen the muscles that surround the painful joint in an effort to increase its inherent stability. For many patients this relieves the pain. The whole concept depends on the joint having lots of big muscles surrounding it to strengthen and provide additional stability. This works well for the lumbar spine in the low back, the knee, and shoulder. For the sacroiliac joint, it is frequently a different story. Because there are no large muscle structures directly crossing the sacroiliac joint, it is difficult to add enough strength to shore up loose and injured ligaments. Laurie's physical therapist provided her a great gift by identifying where her pain was coming from, and although he had helped many patients with chronic SIJ pain, he had not been able to cure her.

The next step for Laurie, like many chronic pain patients with nowhere else to go, was the pain clinic. Not aware of any surgeries that might be of benefit, her primary care doctor sent her to this only remaining source for treatment and a potential cure. She met a female physiatrist there who specialized in chronic pain management. She, like the physical therapist, was adept at diagnosing the sacroiliac joint as a pain center, but unlike the P.T., was able to provide Laure with ongoing viable treatment. Just like thousands of pain doctors across America and around the world, she knew that by injecting an anesthetic and steroid into the joint, she would most likely provide Laurie with some temporary relief, and the remote chance of ending her suffering for good. Laurie began receiving injections, which verified without question that the sacroiliac joint was her pain generator and gave her, each time, a few weeks of significantly reduced pain. This went on for more than two years. Yet, as happens with many types of medication treatment for chronic pain, these injections eventually began to have less effect. Frustrated and miserable, Laurie found herself back at the starting gate.

When someone is trapped in an envelope of chronic pain for many years, more often than not, hopelessness begins to take over. Emotional and mental strength starts to diminish. Just as the body can start to die when deprived of air or food, our inner fortitude can also be worn down, leaving only loss of hope and despair. Inner strength and sense of self-worth can whither away long before the corporal body. We see this too often in news reports and photographs from around the world, where so many live in poverty, fear or oppression, and who, although they are physically alive, reflect in their eyes the hollowness of desolation. Those with disabling sacroiliac joint pain can also, under the right circumstances, end up this way. If we can even contemplate such a person's existence for a only a moment, we can perhaps begin to imagine the depths of this depression.

Laurie told me her pain was worse than what she had endured during the difficult labor and delivery of her son. I was to hear the same from many mothers during the ensuing years. It affected every daily activity; walking, sitting, standing, lying down, sleeping - and each and every one of necessary day-to-day chores. Sex had become a major issue. The physical movements involved, such as abduction of the hips when legs are spread apart, let alone the actual act which impacted the joint repeatedly and felt like being hit inside by a sledgehammer became unbearable. Consequently, there was less and less intimacy between Laurie and her husband. He was becoming frustrated with her. In turn, she felt worthless and misunderstood, which only added to her loss of self-esteem and pushed her further into the depths of despair.

Laurie made up her mind to do whatever it took to save her from the painful life she was living. She didn't know exactly what this would involve, but just making this decision helped empower her and gave her a glimpse of hope. She was a prime example of someone who felt like they had already lost everything, and by making a conscious choice to fight and overcome any obstacles in her mission to find a new direction, she ignited a spark of her remaining inherent strength. Although she had little computer experience, she taught herself to use the Internet and began by searching topics like "chronic pain," "low back pain," and "sacroiliac joint". The more she read about fusion surgery, the more she began to realize this might actually be a solution, and her sense of hope that things could get better returned. She presented this information to her long-time pain doctor and asked her opinion on the chances that fusion might relieve her pain. The doctor was honest with Laurie, admitting she knew little about the procedure, and even that it had gotten a "bad rap" in professional circles. Nevertheless, at Laurie's request, she obliged and made the referral to me.

Up to this point my patients were basically encouraged to see me by professionals and previous patients. Laurie was the first to seek me out on her own, with no one else advocating for her. She had to draw upon her own strength and determination to end up in my office. She had no idea, other than what she had found online, if I was any good, a quack, or just someone who would fail her again. What I saw in her eyes and her demeanor was a weary but strong will that seemed to guide her every step along this uncertain journey.

Laurie was religious and she had turned herself over to her God in this quest to be physically healed so she could live a healthy lifestyle for herself and her family. She also had made up her mind to accept whatever the outcome was to be. She was like someone on a pilgrimage.

For a physician, meeting someone like this who seems to be handing you their body and soul, can be overwhelming. As a doctor, you are immediately in the position of either generating life or taking it away, depending on how you choose to handle the situation. My first reaction was to feel inadequate. I did know that my experience with this joint was growing rapidly, and I wanted very much to help Laurie. Her level of anxiety and desperation as a result of living so long in such pain reminded me not only of the first patient whose sacroiliac joint I had fused, but dozens who had come after. Since my first sacroiliac joint fusion experience, I had the opportunity to meet with, examine, and operate on many individuals who were suffering from both physical and emotional ramifications associated with this joint. Many had disabilities that made their lives nearly impossible, along with relationship problems, financial woes and having to deal with our frustrating medical system. Many of these people were unemployed or unemployable, disabled, on Social Security, and had lawyers trying to carve out an existence for them. Several of my spine surgeon colleagues seemed to find it easy to judge such patients. Early in my surgical practice, I was guilty of that too. There is nothing worse then a judgmental surgeon. He or she tends to listen very little to what they are being told. They may look at their patient almost as an adversary; make quick, rash decisions about a diagnosis and treatment plan, all the while secretly wishing this person was somewhere else.

What brought about a change in my attitude was getting to know these patients, but before that could be meaningful there was a critical decision I needed to make to open the door and allow this to happen. I simply chose to believe what my patients told me about their pain was true. Unfortunately, to do this in the American medical system concerning patients with chronic pain required stepping out of that "know-it-all" box and allowing some vulnerability on both sides. Doing this one thing immediately and for the rest of my career removed a huge weight from my shoulders. I had not realized how heavy a burden it had been to continuously question someone's integrity, assemble facts and fiction about them, constantly wonder if they were being honest, and then come up with my best judgment call. But once I opened myself to simply accept what I was hearing, all of those chains I was dragging around fell away. Suddenly I could concentrate on what each person was saying, and propose what I genuinely felt to be the best treatment. I was now relating to these folks much as I would to my own family. I learned that by directly looking into the eyes of someone who is suffering and allowing yourself to be receptive, you can embrace a sense of vulnerability and truly comprehend not only their suffering, but your own. When you listen with your ears wide open to such people, a bond starts to form. If you are able to think and really try to understand their situation and the hurt they are experiencing, not only physically, but emotionally and spiritually as well, you then might develop real compassion.

I think the wisest and most self-actualized doctors walk away from honest encounters with suffering patients feeling that they received more on a personal and emotional level than did the patient. In the most fruitful doctor-patient relationships healing goes both ways. Patients who build rapport with their doctors can be some of the most compassionate folks you'll ever encounter. Usually, when someone shows compassion to them, they in turn, want to give it back. As a doctor you are expected by nearly everyone to be the steadfast rock of knowledge and deliverance. In reality doctors are just humans and suffer like everyone else. Sometimes it takes patients who have learned to endure their particular malady and are willing to be truly candid, who can open the door for the doctor to learn to do the same thing on a personal level. I had learned this important lesson by the time I met Laurie.

I chose to show Laurie compassion by believing every word of her story and trying to sense how she had suffered, while attempting to find relief through the medical system. I recommended a diagnostic injection into her sacroiliac joint. This was a very positive test that confirmed her pain was indeed coming from that joint. After having only a few days of pain relief from that injection, I subsequently recommended a surgical fusion. Following this course of treatment, Laurie became essentially pain-free and eventually reassumed all of her usual activities, including non-painful sex.

Laurie went on to become an advocate for other sacroiliac joint pain patients. She chose to give back to the suffering community by making herself available to talk to similar patients just getting started on the journey she had endured. Was her pain completely gone? No. But she was certainly happy and satisfied with her long-term results.

I learned a great deal from my interactions with Laurie. I saw just how difficult it was for a patient with chronically disabling sacroiliac joint pain to be understood and appropriately treated by the medical/surgical system. I saw that Laurie's journey had been not only a physical one but a spiritual one as well; during which she turned everything over and admitted she was not in control. She had made the difficult, conscious decision to accept whatever the end result might be. Once her prayers had been answered, she didn't just return to her private life. She chose to share her experience as a way of demonstrating her tremendous gratitude. Laurie's case made me realize that the little world I had been creating was much bigger than I had allowed myself to imagine. I was beginning to understand that this was a universal problem, not limited to my hometown.

Being Your Own Advocate
Lessons from Laurie

1 Sexual intercourse for a woman can result in severe pain if she has a dysfunctional sacroiliac joint. This can lead to avoidance behavior and affect her relationships and self-esteem. Severe chronic sacroiliac joint pain can be equal to or worse than childbirth according to women having experienced both.

2 If you have "hypermobile joints" or are able to dislocate a shoulder or hip joint, you could have lax ligaments and joint capsules holding your sacroiliac joints together, making them more prone to injury and pain. A typical time injury might occur is during child birth.

3 A physical therapist is very good at making the diagnosis of a painful sacroiliac joint, but, in some cases, might not be able to cure the pain.

4 It is important to understand when conservative treatments are not working and seek a referral to an interested surgeon. PTs have, in my experience, been willing to do this, and they usually know the good and interested surgeons.

5 It is important for you to do some research, and the Internet is a good resource. Find a respected surgeon, who is not only interested in this joint but has done some teaching and research on the subject as well.

6 Your journey to find pain relief within America's health care system can be very frustrating and at times feel like a pilgrimage.

7 If your journey is successful and you do receive relief from your chronic sacroiliac joint pain, do what you can to give back and help others on the same journey.

Chapter 4

The Physical Therapist

How a physical therapist with a unique medical history led to an important discovery, and the role arthritis plays in chronic joint pain.

Andrew was different from my other patients in two major respects. First of all, he was a guy. The majority of sacroiliac joint patients are women. Whether this is because they are more prone to this condition or because men are less likely to seek professional help has not been verified. The second distinction was that Andrew was a physical therapist living in a major city, much bigger than the one in which I was practicing. This carried immediate relevance as he was a highly educated professional who had a musculoskeletal problem that was causing him disabling pain, yet could not find the treatment he needed in a large, metropolitan city.

He had located me from my work on the Internet and had then set up an appointment. His story about previous treatments for his low back pain was a significant eye-opener for me, which, like lessons I had learned from other patients, would once again influence how I would proceed with these issues in the future.

Andrew's pain had started years earlier and seemed to come out of nowhere. Thinking that it was probably his lumbar spine he began self-treatment, as most of us professionals do, by stretching and strengthening the muscles in and around that area. This did help at first but over time had less effect. At one point he visited an orthopedic surgeon, whose patients he worked with in his own P.T. practice. Since he had already put himself through all the appropriate conservative therapies for chronic low back pain, his surgeon tried some anti-inflammatory medications, which also helped for a short period of time but then became useless.

Following an MRI and a CT scan of his lumbar spine (or lower back), the surgeon recommended a fusion procedure. Andrew was not the type of person who took a surgical recommendation lightly, so he obtained a second opinion from another orthopedic surgeon. Because both ultimately agreed on his diagnosis and surgical plan, Andrew underwent a lumbar sacral fusion of the two lowest lumbar vertebrae and the sacrum. But six months later he was still experiencing the same severe low back pain. At a loss, Andrew returned to his orthopedist, searching for answers. The surgeon, also frustrated and wanting to help, ordered multiple tests including a CT scan of the fusion area. These tests came back showing that the fusion looked perfect, the instrumentation appropriately placed, and could find no apparent reason for pain in or above that area.

Andrew was becoming truly disheartened. He was essentially being told the pain in his low back had no identifiable cause and subsequently no plan of treatment. He found himself in the same shoes as a lot of his own failed back surgery patients. His surgeon, believing there was nothing further he could do, referred Andrew to the local pain clinic.

Andrew was definitely drifting toward the degree of hopelessness I had seen in so many people suffering from this unrelenting condition. We would soon verify that his pain was emanating from his sacroiliac joint, but meanwhile, he was being misdiagnosed by his surgeon, who simply had not been educated to identify this pain generator. The fault here lay not with the surgeon, but with the entire medical system that inadequately educates physicians how to perform surgery on this joint.

Andrew still felt he was missing something, and by now questioned his ability to be objective about his own diagnosis. So, he asked another physical therapist to evaluate him. It was this therapist who convinced him his pain was most likely connected to his sacroiliac joints.

After a short time he too strongly suspected that his sacroiliac joints were indeed the culprits behind his pain. He had given the same diagnosis to hundreds of his own patients, after utilizing multiple hands-on testing methods that had been passed down through generations of manual clinicians. The wealth of diagnostic knowledge concerning sacroiliac joint pain among physical therapists, chiropractors, and osteopaths at that time was enormous. They knew how to manually test patients and identify a dysfunctional sacroiliac joint. They also knew something else. If they could not resolve a pain crisis using all conservative measures that had stood the test of time, these patients were likely doomed to suffer with no resolution in sight, and their final stopping point would be a chronic pain clinic. Many of these clinicians and doctors did not consider referring a patient for surgical consultation, as that was simply not part of their training.

The pain doctor Andrew subsequently chose to work with agreed to injections to his sacroiliac joints in an effort to first diagnose if these were the pain generators, and secondly to attempt to permanently remove the pain. The first set of injections completely removed Andrew's pain, but only for about 3 hours. This did at least validate that his pain was originating from those joints. However, after two weeks the pain was back, severe as ever. A second set of injections was performed with almost the exact same result, no pain for the first three hours, then returning to full fervor by the one-week mark.

Thousands of individuals today find themselves in this exact same situation, as they work with pain doctors to treat their chronic sacroiliac joint pain. Each set of injections verifies that, yep, the problem is the sacroiliac joint, and although they seem to help for a brief period, eventually severe pain returns and the process starts all over again. Andrew thus found himself caught in the "revolving door" of ongoing injection management for what had now developed into crippling pain. But he was not willing to accept this as a final option. He had the advantage of actually knowing more about these joints than his pain doctor, so he requested a referral to someone who performed sacroiliac surgeries on a regular basis. Andrew's doctor was a reasonable fellow who agreed that fusion of both sacroiliac joints was probably the only likely solution left. He then referred him back to the orthopedic surgeon who had performed his lumbosacral fusion. After running more tests on the previous fusion area to be sure nothing had been overlooked, the surgeon concurred that sacroiliac joint fusions were probably in order. He went on to say that, like most orthopedic surgeons of that time, he had little experience in fusing this joint and had only performed this surgery in trauma situations using the 'two screws across the joint" method. Although these surgeries did stabilize the joint, they did little to relieve pain. He told Andrew that if he could find someone who was experienced in performing fusions for this purpose, he would be happy to refer him.

By the time Andrew showed up in my office I had performed over 100 fusions for the sacroiliac joint, and within the medical/surgical system I might as well have been the "Lone Ranger." As far as I knew there were only about four surgeons in America who really understood this joint and the severe disabling pain it could cause, that a significant number of conservative treatments fail, and that various types of sacroiliac joint fusions had proven to have a high likelihood of relieving pain. At the time there was still no mention of or education for this painful condition by the medical and surgical educational societies anywhere.

Unlike most patients, because of all Andrew had been through, he required no further work-up on my part and could be put immediately on the surgery schedule. He was also my first patient to require bilateral sacroiliac joint fusions after having had a perfectly performed and well-healed lumbosacral fusion. This compelled me to start looking into what factors led to chronically painful sacroiliac joints. Andrew's unique medical history of having had a previous L4-S1 lumbosacral fusion would eventually, through bench and clinical research, lead to the discovery that such a fusion can be one of the primary causes for needing a sacroiliac joint fusion at a later date. This is due to the fact that the sacroiliac joint pain was initially missed as a pain generator or the lumbar fusion put extra stress on the joint. The following two paragraphs summarize my experience with these causes for chronic sacroiliac joint pain as I discussed in the 2015 textbook, *"Surgery for the painful sacroiliac joint: a clinical guide"* **(ref 6)**.

The bench, or lab research I discuss in this book consisted of a simulation of Andrew's fusion, and used cadaver specimens to test range of motion of the sacroiliac joint after rigidly stabilizing the lowest level of the lumbar sacral spine. Results showed that stresses on the sacroiliac joint were much greater when the lower part of the lumbar sacral spine was prevented from moving. This made sense, as in any structure where there are two or more moving parts, if you immobilize one, the others are placed under increased pressure.

The clinical research that I later performed on 99 consecutive patients with sacroiliac joint fusions at our institution, and which I had followed for almost 4 years, revealed that 65% had previous lumbosacral fusions prior to their diagnosis of sacroiliac joint pain. Andrew was fortunate because his fusion was appropriately performed from a technical aspect and was solid. Many others were not so lucky. More than two thirds continued to suffer because they either did not have solid fusions or had other degenerative arthritis changes occurring above or below the lumbosacral fusion. In these cases, if pain generators in the sacroiliac joints and the spine were not both addressed during fusion surgery, there would be residual pain from whichever one was not treated.

As I evaluated my patient population for various pathological causes for chronic sacroiliac joint pain, it became clear that it all boiled down to some form of arthritis. What is it about arthritis that generates pain? The place to start is to define what arthritis is in a human. The origin of the word arthritis comes from two words, "arthro," which means joint, or a movable area between two bones, and "itis," which means inflammation. There are two types of arthritis that we as Homo sapiens experience, both of which can lead to chronic pain. Osteoarthritis is the garden-variety type that grandpa has in his hip or knee. Inflammatory arthritis can include rheumatoid, lupus and many other varieties. The difference between the two is like night and day.

In osteoarthritis, cartilage, or the glistening surface between two bones, begins to erode and the bone it is attached to (subchondral bone) has to assume more and more stress. The body reacts by attempting to fuse the joint on its own by laying down extra bone (spurs) around the joint in an attempt to stop all motion and prohibit the eroding process. Osteoarthritis is caused by multiple factors, but genetics has been shown to be one of the most important. The saying, "Like father, like son," is unfortunately very apt with this condition. The average total hip or knee replacement is performed due to this type of arthritis.

With inflammatory arthritis, a person's own blood cells, those used to fight infection or foreign bodies, attack their own joints. This "attack," in its worst-case scenario, can be vicious and unrelenting. The cells seek and destroy joint tissues much like acid can consume flesh. After leaving a joint utterly decimated, the chemicals released by the invading cells erode into the bone, break through the joint capsules, and can attack surrounding ligaments and tendons. This can mean severe crippling, pain and deformities **(Fig 5)**.

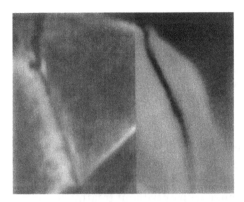

Fig 5. The CT scan cross section on the left shows that with inflammatory arthritis the joint line is pitted from the erosive chemical reactions from one's own cells. On the right the joint line remains smooth, illustrating that with degeneration of the cartilage the bone beneath becomes more dense to withstand increased stresses.

The crucial factor, about which I have published research, suggests that fusing an osteoarthritic, chronically painful sacroiliac joint can effect considerable relief, whereas fusing the same joint affected by inflammatory arthritis might not have the same beneficial effect. The reasons for this difference are currently unknown.

Many conditions can lead to osteoarthritis of the sacroiliac joint. The most common, as in Andrew's case, is a previous lumbar sacral fusion, which increases the stresses on those joints. In Andrew's particular case his pain was the same, or worse, after his low back fusion suggesting that it may have been in his sacroiliac joints all along. If this was the case, his low back fusion actually could have resulted in those joints generating actually more pain. Trauma, such as from an automobile or motorcycle accident is another common cause, followed by falls from a height. It can even come about just falling from a standing position onto the buttock.

Sometimes, osteoarthritis in this joint is due to a condition one is born with, like a Type IIa or IIb lumbosacral vertebral segment (LSTV), where the lowest lumbar vertebrae and the sacrum are under-or over-developed. Orthopedic spine surgeons are taught and tested on this condition, but are not trained as to how it relates to chronic sacroiliac joint pain. Osteoarthritis can also develop after an over-zealous attempt to harvest bone graft from the pelvic bone, usually for spine surgery. This typically happens due to a traumatic impact to the joint itself, or by the simple act of removing some of the supporting ligaments in the process.

Every now and then the sacroiliac joint can become infected, either from normal bacteria circulating in the blood stream and lodging in the surrounding bone capillaries, or after an injection. Once the infection runs its course with or without treatment, the joint can be left with inadequate and damaged anatomy that may evolve into severe degenerative arthritis. The same thing can happen when acute swelling of the joint from inflammatory arthritis recedes, and what's left of the tissue continues to degenerate. The majority of patients who undergo surgery for fusion of this joint have arthritic changes that provoke pain when stressed in any way. A major distinction between this type of painful sacroiliac joint and one that is due to acute trauma is that the former is usually very stable, while the latter is extremely unstable. The inherent stability in an arthritic sacroiliac is one of two reasons it is difficult for orthopedic surgeons to accept it is a pain generator.

Surgeons dealing with chronic pain from a joint have known for over a century that if an arthritic joint, which has lots of motion, is fused together, pain relief is very likely. For instance, before total hip or knee replacements were available, it was necessary for an orthopedic surgeon to fuse the joint together to stop the motion and thus the pain. In those days, this was a difficult surgical task, especially for the hip joint, but, if accomplished, usually was successful. The first recorded fusion of two bones, which I mentioned earlier, did not occur until the late 1800s. That particular fusion was of the knee joint. Today we just put in a totally new mechanical knee or hip, which not only relieves pain but also maintains the motion of the joint. The sacroiliac joint presents an entirely different perspective in terms of pain resulting from joint instability and severe arthritis.

The mindset of an orthopedic surgeon regarding the sacroiliac joint has historically been that if it is grossly unstable (actively moves a centimeter or more with applied pressure), it can be painful. Two examples of this, which I learned in medical school and residency, are a traumatic separation of the sacroiliac joint, say from a car accident or fall, and the laxity and separation which occurs in the last trimester of pregnancy, which continues for two to three months after a vaginal delivery. Both can bring about severe pain. What happens to this logical thinking when a surgeon is looking at an X-Ray of a very stable sacroiliac joint that may or may not have arthritis, in a patient suffering from severe chronic pain? Suddenly it is not so logical. If you add to the mix that it has now been proven that the actual movement of this joint during daily activities is only about one or two degrees, and almost non-detectable, it further confuses the picture. Why does this very stable joint that very often has minimal to no observable arthritis cause disabling pain? What and where exactly is the pain source? The answers to both of these questions are a big "we don't know"! And yet we can see in hundreds of cases, like Andrew's, where surgical fusion for pain associated with stable sacroiliac joints results in frequently less or no pain afterward.

One of the major reasons that medical schools and institutions of higher learning for orthopedic and neurosurgeons does not teach surgical solutions for chronic sacroiliac joint pain possibly results from the lack of instability and arthritis that these joints demonstrate. Put another way, it is hard to teach about fusing something together that looks and acts pretty stable.

Andrew, who had very stable sacroiliac joints with minimal to no obvious arthritis, went on to have surgery, which fused both of his sacroiliac joints. He was a model patient, trusting his diagnosis and having faith that he would resume a normal life after a period of healing and rehabilitation. He did indeed do well, and several years later said unequivocally that he was extremely satisfied with his decision and the results of his surgery. Andrew reinforced for me the fact that the sacroiliac joint does cause severe disabling pain in certain people, and that patients like him who typically do not have his level of knowledge feel very lost and alone. He taught me that it takes strong motivation to keep searching for answers in a society not well informed on the subject, and that it is essential to trust the person who may actually have answers needed to move forward. Andrew also made me realize once and for all that people should not have to suffer with severe disabling pain from a sacroiliac joint in this day and age.

Being Your Own Advocate
Lessons from Andrew

1 Both men and women can suffer from chronic sacroiliac joint pain.

2 This chronic pain can be in both joints, and each could need a surgical solution.

3 The lower spinal bones, "lumbar vertebrae", could be mistaken as the source of low back pain, when in fact it is coming from the sacroiliac joints.

4 If your surgeon does not understand surgery for the sacroiliac joints, use whatever means you can (e.g. Internet) to find one who does.

5 Both sacroiliac joints can be fused at the same time. If your surgeon uses a lateral minimally invasive approach there could be a long period of minimal weight bearing for both lower extremities. I used the procedure discussed in ref. 6 to perform dozens of bilateral sacroiliac joint fusions, which allowed for full weight bearing immediately after surgery.

6 When a specific cause is found to explain chronic sacroiliac joint pain, it is frequently a form of arthritis. Keep in mind that the sacroiliac joint can be very painful and debilitating even when there is no obvious arthritis present on imaging studies. The scientific reason for this is currently unknown.

7 You don't have to continue to suffer with chronic sacroiliac joint pain in this day and age. This may require some very proactive steps on your part.

Chapter 5
Wake- Up Call

Even a successful surgery can have surprising and serious complications.

When Betsy came to see me she was a single mom in her mid forties, a thin, wiry woman with tremendous energy. Some sort of physical expression accentuated everything she said. She was like a force of nature, the type of person who wasn't afraid to take on anything, without any doubt she would succeed. But her message was clear. She had been living every day with intense low back pain and she'd had enough! She was ready to dive into anything that might promise relief.

Betsy was from a small rural town about a hundred miles north of Kalamazoo, Michigan, where she had grown up as an only child without a father. She and her mother worked whatever jobs they could find to make ends meet and continued to live together in the same small house in which she had been born. Together, they were a dynamic duo and dealt with whatever life threw at them. Though Betsy had dropped out of school before finishing high school, she had more on the ball than many college graduates, and knew how to navigate through life. She was a survivor.

Betsy had suffered from severe pain for more than two years by the time I met her. It was her physical therapist who sent her my way, thinking the cause was very likely her sacroiliac joint.

I did not know at the time of our first meeting that Betsy would be someone who would advance my overall knowledge about problems, which can occur as a result of sacroiliac joint fusion surgery. Of course, before each surgery I went over all potential complications with each patient. But somehow (probably as a result of having performed several hundreds of these procedures with no residual issues), I had come to expect nothing life threatening, and on some level believed that my patients were immune to any adverse effects. Betsy's diagnosis and the decision to perform a fusion of her sacroiliac joint were as straightforward as it could possibly be. Her pain was in exactly the right place, a long trial of physical therapy had failed to relieve it, and the diagnostic injection verified that her pain was coming from that joint. After looking diligently for any other sources, I was confident that the cause was definitely her right sacroiliac joint. We discussed the option of surgery; all the pros and cons, including the possibility of critical (but remote) complications. Betsy was 100% on board to move ahead. The sooner the better as far as she was concerned.

If I were asked to pick the one sacroiliac joint fusion of my entire career that I thought was as classic as they could come, it would be Betsy's. It went like clockwork, and she was up on her feet and walking the very next morning. She was so happy, because the severe pain she had been suffering for so long was gone. There was normal post-operative pain to deal with, but, for Betsy, that was nothing compared to the unrelenting pain she'd been enduring. She went home 24 hours later and continued to improve her mobility and grow stronger. Her activity restrictions for the first six weeks following surgery were simple; she was not to lift more than ten pounds and needed to limit bending and twisting at her waist. She was to walk as much as she could tolerate, using a shorter stride to keep stress off the fusion site. I can honestly say that when she left the hospital I thought she was home free and would do very well.

But, life can prove unpredictable. Often, when we think we have our future all planned and thought out, inevitably the rug gets pulled out from under us. Such was Betsy's experience.

About two weeks after her surgery, a doctor in the emergency room at the hospital in her small town contacted me. Betsy had come into their E.R. by ambulance, with severe chest pain and almost unable to breath. After putting her on oxygen and stabilizing her, they performed numerous tests. All of them ultimately showed that what had caused the chest pain and labored breathing was a blood clot that had migrated up from her leg and lodged in one of her lungs. The medical term for this is a "pulmonary embolism," which in some cases can be fatal.

I couldn't have been more shocked when I heard this news about Betsy. Of all people, it seemed incredible that this could happen to someone who not only had undergone an operation as close to perfect as possible, but who possessed such a strong will and confidence that everything would work out for the best no matter what.

Betsy could have died that day. Death from a blood clot can happen very quickly once it has lodged in a lung. But clots can be deceptive. They range from very small clots, which block the tinier vessels and go undetected, to much larger ones, blocking major vessels, in which case they can cause instant death. There is no way to predict such an event, but those who don't die immediately and are fortunate enough to make it to the emergency room in time can be saved.

A blood clot developing in the leg, usually the calf area, is a complication well known to orthopedic surgeons. It occurs most commonly in people who have been through a traumatic event like a car accident and have broken bones, especially in the legs or pelvis. When a clot forms, for many reasons beyond the scope of this book, it can sometime dislodge and float up through the veins on its way toward the lungs. If you think of the blood vessels of the lung like the branches of a tree, you can visualize how the vessels start out big, like a tree trunk, then slowly branch off and expand into clusters of tiny vessels. It is at the very tips of these clusters that oxygen from the lungs enters the blood cells. In Betsy's case, although a sizable section of her lung was blocked, it was not enough to kill her. Her treatment then called for intravenous medication to thin her blood, which helps prevent more clots from developing. The original clot then slowly is dissolved by the body's own defenses thus increasing the lungs ability to work normally again.

Through encounters with trauma patients, surgeons have long understood blood clots and their propensity to create pulmonary embolisms. As we began to perform more and more elective surgeries to put in new hip joints and knee joints we learned that they could occur after those surgeries as well. The research is not definitive, but all in all there is a 1-5% chance of a blood clot developing in the leg after such a procedure. When Betsy had her pulmonary embolism, following an elective and very routine, uncomplicated sacroiliac joint fusion it was definitely an eye-opener and "wake-up" call for me.

Betsy's almost disastrous event gave me pause. It forced me to re-evaluate my expectations that nothing was likely to go wrong, especially in the most routine procedures. I was reminded that no matter how well surgeries are performed, the unexpected can still occur. Although there was no way in which I could have predicted her pulmonary embolism, after Betsy's near-death experience I made an even more conscious effort to spend as much time as necessary, thoroughly explaining all possible risks to ensure my patients were completely informed, regardless of how routine their procedure appeared to be. It was important that I, as a surgeon, along with my patients, never took any surgery for granted. After experiencing her case I began to instruct my patients to take a baby aspirin each day after surgery to slightly thin the blood and possibly prevent a clot in the leg from developing. It also reinforced to me how diligent the rehabilitation process needs to be, especially being up and walking after surgery to keep the blood in the legs flowing.

A few weeks later Betsy returned for a follow-up exam. She was recovering well and seemed once again to be her usual happy, animated self. She had no pain in her chest or low back. She went on to fully rehabilitate and back to living a life full of energy and free from pain.

I learned a lot from Betsy. Not only did she reaffirm that every sacroiliac joint fusion surgery was a major operation with serious potential complications, she taught me how one could take an adverse life event in stride while maintaining a very positive attitude along the way. She was amazing! And, once again, I was reminded that I was not in total control, and my faith in the wonder and awe of life and living was again reignited.

Being Your Own Advocate
Lessons from Betsy

1 Having a seemingly simple sacroiliac joint fusion is, in reality, a major operation having potential for major complications, which, although very rare, can be life threatening.

2 Your surgeon should explain in detail all the potential complications and their relative risks regardless of how rare or remote.

3 If you feel that you have not received enough information about your surgery, do not hesitate to ask more questions. Several potential questions are listed in the chapter "The Sacrolllac Joint Playbook".

4 Maintaining an attitude of hope, joy, and gratitude is one of the best forms of "self-care".

Chapter 6
Double Jeopardy

Why surgeons should always consider the spine and sacroiliac joints as possible dual pain generators.

The mood in the exam room where Sharon and her husband waited was sullen and gloomy as I walked in. Nine years ago, I had performed Sharon's two-level lumbosacral spine fusion and since then she had been managing very well. After her initial surgery, she had fully recovered and subsequently returned to a very busy lifestyle.

Sharon had now come back to see me because the pain in her low back had begun to reoccur within the past year, accompanied by new pain shooting down her legs. It had gotten so severe that she could no longer do many of the things that made her happiest. She wasn't able to play with and enjoy her two young grandsons. She and her husband loved to travel and had been all over the world, but now she couldn't keep up with him. Her full and active life had ground to a standstill. The woman I remembered as animated and always full of life and laughter was sitting in front of me looking miserable and despondent.

I watched as she sat silently next to her husband, all curled up, arms wrapped around her. Barely holding back tears, she finally mumbled something, which I struggled to understand. Even though I couldn't hear her exact words, it was obvious that she was in much worse pain than when I had first seen her years before.

Sharon's original surgery had involved attaching two titanium rods to her spine with six pedicle screws, and bone graft from her pelvic bone, which spanned the two lowest spinal segments in her low back. At this point, with the cause of her current pain unknown, my immediate concern was that something had gone wrong as a result of her previous fusion. However, the last time I had seen her, at her last surgical follow up exam, X-Rays of the entire site had looked good. That procedure had worked well, and kept her pain-free for almost a decade. The pains she had now were not located in the same area as her previous fusion.

One painful spot seemed just above her previous back incision, the other just below it. She had no pain in the area over her incision, which was the site of the fusion. I knew right away that trying to figure out where these latest pains were originating was going to take a complicated work-up.

Sharon was now in her late fifties, but still wanted to be as active as possible. She and her husband were both visibly frightened, as though expecting a verdict they did not want to hear. My gut feeling was that they might be right, and that their lives may be about to change significantly.

During the next several days Sharon went through multiple tests in an effort to find out what was generating her pain and why. These included CT scans, X-Rays, and injections, after which her diagnoses finally became clear. First of all, her previous surgery looked fine; nothing had moved or broken. As explained earlier, if part of the spine is fused, or made solid, the stresses can increase on either side of that fusion during normal movements of daily living. That is exactly what was happening with Sharon. The two vertebrae, or spinal segments, above her two-level fusion had developed severe arthritis due to increased stresses placed on them from the original fusion. One of these boney vertebra had loosened and was slipping or moving inappropriately whenever she bent her back. The other issue was that the nerves inside these spinal segments were being pinched by the arthritis. This happens when arthritis builds up inside the spinal canal, narrowing the space nerves go through and generating nerve pain, which can radiate down the legs, making the whole situation more disabling. The pain from these vertebrae and the nerves involved was going on above her previous fusion. For the same reasons; increasing stresses and arthritis, both her sacroiliac joints had become sources for severe pain below her previous fusion. This particular situation meant that Sharon was having severe disabling pain coming from both the spine and the sacroiliac joints at the same time. The logic here is that in order to relieve her pain, both areas had to be treated.

Since the time I had first met Sharon and performed her low back fusion, I had experienced a significant number of patients caught in this predicament. I decided to research them as a group, and in 2015 published a paper discussing outcomes when both areas of pain generation, the spine and sacroiliac joints, were fused at the same time. I then compared this group to previous studies published in medical literature by others, where only *one* of the two pain generating areas was fused **(ref 7)**. The results showed that in those patients who had both areas fused, long-term success rates were much higher, in one comparison as much as 69%. As this book goes to press, this remains the only study published in world literature that considers both the sacroiliac joints and the lower spine as pain generators being fused at the same setting and the resulting long-term outcomes. It is also the only research offering a surgical option for patients with this type of dual pain. At some point in the future it will become clear to orthopedic surgeons and neurosurgeons that this dual pain pathology exists, and that both areas need to be treated in order to obtain the best result for pain relief.

After appropriate testing that confirmed the pain was coming from both of these areas, Sharon and her husband appeared to completely understand her situation. I explained to them that I could operate on one of the two areas and see if the other needed to be done, but I had been down that road many times in the past. Each time I inevitably ended up coming back to perform the fusion of the other pain generator. Over time I evolved to performing both fusions at the same setting and the overall results improved.

Sharon's next surgery consisted of removing the instrumentation that had been used in her previous lower spine operation, extending the fusion several levels up her spine after opening up the space in the spinal canal that was pinching the nerves going into her legs, and fusing both sacroiliac joints together. She went on to have a successful recovery and, at her long-term follow-up exam 4 years later, said she was able to enjoy many of the activities she had thought would never be possible again.

Being Your Own Advocate
Lessons from Sharon

1 Pain generators that are disabling can be in the lower spine and the sacroiliac joints at the same time.

2 In order to effectively treat or cure the chronic pain under these circumstances, both areas must be diagnosed and treated.

3 It is up to you to ask your surgeon if this is, or is not, the situation in your particular case, as there is no formal education for your surgeon to be considering this as a possibility. Those surgeons who understand it have somehow stumbled on this concept through their own self-education.

Chapter 7
America's Sacroiliac Joint In The New Millennium

Reasons this joint is often overlooked and how to navigate America's health system to find answers.

My experience with so many frustrated, anxious and depressed patients caused me to look deeper into the dilemma of the patient with SI Joint pain, who had nowhere to turn for help.

Why did it seem the educational leaders in orthopedic surgery were being so resistant to proper education and research for the dysfunctional and chronically painful sacroiliac joint? The concept of pain coming from the sacroiliac joint, which has been part of the medical spectrum for a century, had been overshadowed by the long existing and overwhelming knowledge that the lumbar spine in the low back was definitively proven to result in lower back and leg pain. Tens of thousands of articles have verified this for over 70 years and thus it has become for surgeons the only probable pain generator for those areas. Because hundreds of notable orthopedic spine surgeons spent their entire careers working on patients with low back pain resulting from the spine, and not looking outside the spine for other causes, this became the "textbook" reason for this type of pain.

Since it serves many surgeons' egos to look only at successes they have achieved using the same, unchallenged approach (which is especially true amongst the "Old Guard," whose lead many surgeons follow faithfully), their perspective on this has become even more polarized, making this the accepted stance on low back pain and the standard for the entire medical/surgical community. The financial incentive is also strong; every aspect of the lumbar spine that generates pain now has instrumentation designed to treat that condition. This equipment is extremely expensive and, with the insertion of it becoming more minimally invasive, it has been successfully marketed to the masses. This has resulted in continuing huge profits for both industry and surgeons. For surgeons to take the time and energy to learn about pain generated by the sacroiliac joint and understand the physical and emotional toll it can take, would require a paradigm shift, and a complete departure from the complacent and profitable situation into which they have settled.

The chronically painful and dysfunctional sacroiliac joint has been misunderstood throughout the course of the past century. It has gone from being the only reason for low back and leg pain to being displaced by the discovery of the lumbar herniated disc, now rediscovered but without any real consensus or standardization, neither by orthopedic and neurosurgeons, nor their respective educational societies. Those suffering from this condition have had a bumpy ride, to say the least. There are several thousands of others fortunate to have received good surgical treatment after all conservative measures failed, but these success stories are certainly not due to any organized approach by America's health system.

Today, America's medical and surgical establishments are dealing with the sacroiliac joint in ways both good and bad. There are multiple levels within this system; individual doctors, medical educational societies, hospitals and industries, and finally, government agencies in charge of regulating treatments and protecting patients.

The overall perspective on the sacroiliac joint can be traced in part to the fundamental definition of life in our country today, democratic capitalism. Several highly regarded publications over the past three decades estimate that the sacroiliac joint is responsible for low back pain in 15 to 22% of individuals who see a clinician **(refs 1,2,3)**. Some push this up to 30%. The majority of the rest experience pain stemming from the lumbar spine. This has been my experience as well, during thirty years of clinical and surgical practice. Since this information has been widely publicized for many years, one would assume that clinicians of all specialties would routinely look at the SI Joint as a possible diagnosis during their initial exams. It has been well described in recent literature that all a clinician has to do is push on one well-defined spot just above the buttock, which, if it elicits pain, means the sacroiliac joint is the possible source and further testing is needed to rule it in or out as a pain generator **(Fig 6)(ref 8)**.

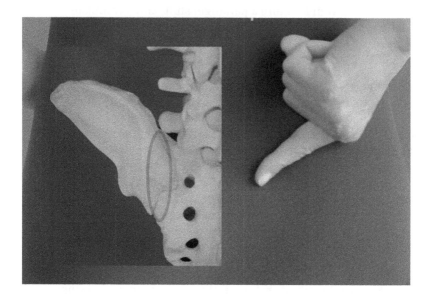

Fig 6. This patient is pointing to the area on the back frequently associated with sacroiliac joint pain. This is an example of the "Fortin Finger Test." Pain in this location indicates the sacroiliac joint may be the pain generator.

Seems simple, right? Wrong! In reality, with the exception of osteopaths, doctors ranging from primary care to orthopedic surgeons and neurosurgeons, who see tens of thousands of these patients each year, do not routinely check for this diagnosis. I too, followed this course until 1991, twelve years after receiving my medical degree and six years after beginning my practice as an orthopedic spine surgeon. I now ask why do we allow this to continue? How could a patient receive proper treatment for chronic low back pain if part of their anatomy that potentially generates severe pain up to 22% of the time is totally overlooked? The answer is complex, and involves elements from many levels within our medical system.

Keep in mind that I am not saying the entire medical system in

America is complicit in this. As I've stated previously, for decades pain doctors, anesthesiologists, physiatrists, chiropractors and physical therapists were all taught how to diagnose severe sacroiliac joint pain, and how to treat it. It is a key area they look at when evaluating a new back pain patient. Each specialty has developed its own way of providing potential relief, and it is roughly estimated that they are successful in treating 80% or more of patients with this diagnosis. All of these clinicians provide some form of conservative care but none perform surgery. The bottom line is that if an individual suffering from this particular problem sees one of these types of clinicians first, and they fall into that 80% success group, life is golden. But what happens to those who first consult an orthopedic or neurosurgeon? Unless those individuals happen to find the rare surgeon who has learned to identify and deal with this joint, how that person will be diagnosed and ultimately treated, both physically and emotionally, is, to put it bluntly, a crapshoot.

One might ask at this point why, when conservative treatments fail, don't clinicians then make a surgical referral? This would seem the logical sequence of events, but the reason it does not often happen is somewhat complicated, and frequently involves money. A physical therapist can only work with a patient for a certain period of time if the treatments are not curative or if the patient is not making significant progress. After that the insurance company simply doesn't pay the therapist. P.T.'s are then likely to recommend a surgical consult, and are actually one of the only type of "pain" clinicians who are primary referral sources for surgeons. Chiropractors and pain clinic doctors, such as anesthesiologists and physiatrists, however, can see a patient literally forever and will continue to be paid whether the patient improves or not. To send such a patient off for definitive surgical treatment would in effect remove a "cash cow" from their practices. In all fairness, they also may not make a referral because they are not trained, just as surgeons are not trained to know that good surgical solutions are available.

This overwhelming lack of surgical education about the sacroiliac joint impacts thousands and thousands of people in the US. During the 1990s and the first seven or eight years of this century, much of the work being done by only a very few orthopedic spine surgeons, who acquired knowledge on their own, or were mentored by surgeons who were self-taught, on the development of surgeries for this joint, used a posterior or posterior lateral approach to perform these fusions. A handful of substantive papers that they managed to publish about these approaches show favorable results for pain relief, with very low complication rates.

By the year 2000 the medical device industry, as a result of working with the few orthopedic surgeons interested in this joint, was beginning to understand that the sacroiliac did cause severe pain and that methods to deal with it needed to be developed. But still, nothing moved forward, for a couple of reasons. The first was that the average orthopedic spine surgeon and neurosurgeon understood very little about this issue and many were reluctant to delve into it further. It was felt that this was an area for orthopedic trauma surgeons, who also did not want to get involved with chronic sacroiliac pain. The other reason was a large roadblock constructed by the Federal Drug Administration (FDA). "Pre-market approval" was needed before implementation of a fusion device using one of the posterior or posterior lateral procedures could proceed. This is the same type of approval process pharmaceutical companies face when developing a new drug. The estimated initial cost can run as high as $70 million, and can take several years of clinical trials to even get such a product to market. Between 2000 and 2008, this industry was unwilling to make such an investment, when major orthopedic and neurosurgical educational societies were essentially ignoring the chronically painful sacroiliac joint and continuing to focus solely on pain pathology in the spine. However, custom devices, those designed for surgeons researching new ways of performing surgery, were being successfully placed into the sacroiliac joint for pain relief. I personally had many successful procedures using a few hundred of these custom devices from a company called Medtronic. These surgeries had been proven effective and safe, as published in prominent peer review journals. Nevertheless, in order for Medtronic and other manufacturers to mass-produce a custom device and teach surgeons how to use it, the FDA pre-market approval was still required. My frustration with the situation was no different from that of the handful of other earnest colleagues scattered across America, each working with industry in the same way I was and attempting to help patients with severe suffering from the sacroiliac joint.

One bright spot during this time was that a standardized method for diagnosing the chronically painful sacroiliac joint, using a certain injection protocol, was finally universally agreed upon and validated in medical literature **(Fig 7)(ref 9)**.

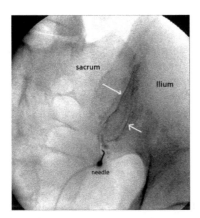

Fig 7. Dye injected into and disseminated throughout the sacroiliac joint (outlined by arrows) is verification that the medications (usually a numbing agent and a steroid) are being placed in the true joint.

In this procedure the sacroiliac joint is injected with both a dye, and medications consisting of a steroid and a numbing agent. The dye confirms that the medications are in the joint. The numbing medication should remove pain generating from the joint for one to four hours depending on the type used. With the steroid, a longer period of pain relief is hoped for as this actually decreases cells believed responsible for causing pain. If an individual has at least a 90% decrease in pain for as long as the numbing medication is expected to last, the pain is determined to be coming from the sacroiliac joint. If there is minimal or no decrease in pain during this time then we can conclude the sacroiliac joint is not causing pain.

This injection protocol opened the door for pain doctors, primarily anesthesiologists and psychiatrists, to begin treating pain in this joint, and diagnosing thousands of patients with chronic severe pain originating from it. Patients could now be accurately diagnosed with this condition for the first time in human history.

Once this news hit the Internet, those sufferers willing to be their own health advocates were able to seek more definitive treatment after conservative approaches had proven ineffective. They could now search for orthopedic or neurosurgeons who were engaged in active research for this painful joint, surgically treating it, and publishing the results. A patient could either attempt to make an appointment with a surgeon directly or obtain a referral through his or her pain doctor, physical therapist, or primary care physician. During this time, over half of my surgical fusion patients found me using this method.

Remember that the diagnosis of chronic sacroiliac joint pain had been in limbo since its re-emergence in the mid-1980s. But in 2008 the dormant world of chronic sacroiliac joint pain was turned on its head. Industry found a way to get around the "pre-market approval" by literally bypassing the FDA altogether. A loophole in FDA regulations allowed an alternative designation. Since the agency was created in 1976, any device proven to be a surgical instrument existing prior to the inception of the FDA was eligible for 510(k) status, which meant it was considered safe and effective, and equivalent to a legal device already being used and not subject to pre-market approval.

In the trauma world of orthopedics, long before the FDA was formed, there existed a situation in which a patient's pelvis could be injured in a fall or automobile accident in such a way that the sacroiliac joint was literally torn apart. This was a violent and destabilizing injury, requiring surgery that would attach the pelvic wing bone back to the sacral bone and re-establish the sacroiliac joint connection. Initially, this was done by making a long incision over the buttock and cutting deeply through very vascularized muscle to place two long screws from the pelvic bone, across the sacroiliac joint, into the sacral bone **(Fig 8)**.

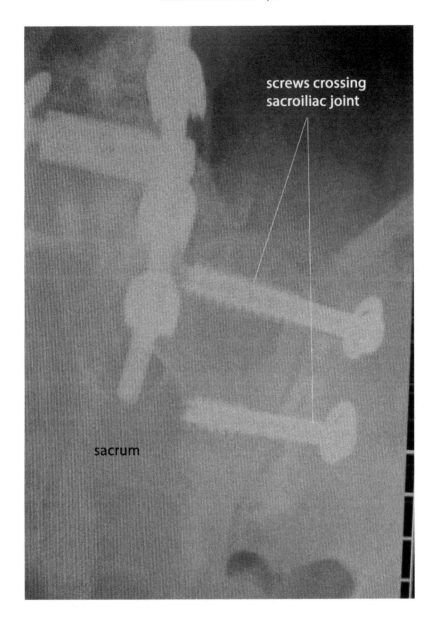

Fig 8. X-Ray of two bone screws being placed across the sacroiliac joint, after trauma pulled it apart, to hold it in proper position. The left side shows instrumentation from a lower spine fusion occurring after sacroiliac joint surgery.

This was a very bloody surgery, but, if there were no complications, usually resulted in holding the sacroiliac joint in place. It is estimated that 50% of these patients continued to have severe pain, which they were forced to live with forever. During the 1970s and 80s the same "two-screw" procedure, as shown in **Fig 8,** was used only occasionally in patients with chronic pain from stable non-traumatized sacroiliac joints, and achieved about the same success rate of a 50% reduction in pain.

Industry was able to create a device that could be inserted using the "pre FDA" techniques and simulate the old "two screws across the joint" procedure, thus making them eligible for 510(k) status. By using an X-Ray machine with continuous radiation, they enabled surgeons to actually see an image showing anatomical landmarks and the precise final position of each piece of hardware being inserted. This resulted in less damage to tissue during the procedure. Since 2008 several companies have developed devices to stabilize or fuse the SIJoint in a much less invasive way than the original procedure handed down long ago by the trauma surgeons **(Fig 9)**.

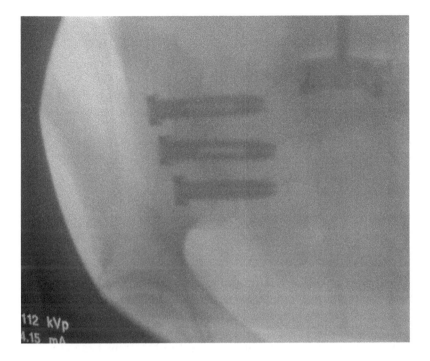

Fig 9. X-Ray of three modern screws crossing the sacroiliac joint, inserted in a minimally invasive approach, through small incisions on the lateral buttock for diagnosis of chronic sacroiliac joint pain.

The 510(k) designation opened the door for FDA approved mass production of surgical devices for fusing sacroiliac joints. As part of their marketing efforts, the makers of these new implements included information about the severe pain associated with a dysfunctional sacroiliac joint, and thus helped increase awareness of this condition among surgeons and the general public.

We now had a surgical approach, along with several device options that actually worked, and patients could finally understand exactly what was causing their pain.

Before long, device manufacturers were profiting, progress was being made, and more surgeries for the painful dysfunctional sacroiliac joint were being performed in America every year. *Becker's Orthopedic & Spine Review* **(ref 10)** (a leading resource for news and analysis on business and legal issues relating to orthopedic and spine practices), reported that [under the 510(k) umbrella], about 8000 sacroiliac joint fusions or stabilization surgeries had been performed in 2014 employing the lateral approach and new devices.

At first glance, this seemed like a major advance in treatment of patients with SI joint pain. But in reality, something far less positive was taking place. Historically, in our medical system the patient had always been the top priority, was of primary importance, and was the beneficiary of both scientific and industrial progress. Putting the patient first in all respects had been the credo and consensus of surgeons, industry and medical educational societies. With the introduction and aggressive marketing of expensive new devices, and the push for profits by manufacturers, this hierarchy began to change.

To help visualize this dramatic shift within our healthcare system, I created the following illustrations, which I refer to as " The Pyramids of Importance."

Most Important

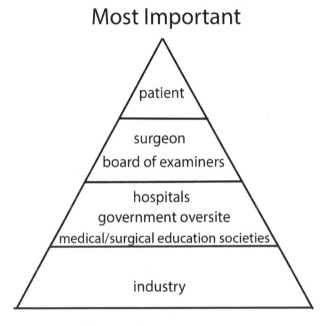

Least Important

Pyramid of importance,
as applies to sacroiliac joint fusion surgery
in 1985

Illustration one

The U.S. Medical System's "Pyramid of Importance" up to 1985, indicating the patient as top priority.

Most Important

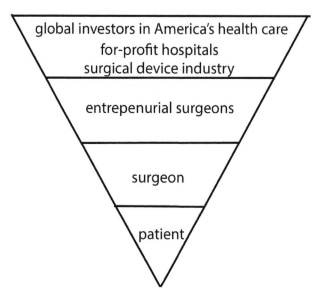

global investors in America's health care
for-profit hospitals
surgical device industry

entrepenurial surgeons

surgeon

patient

Least Important

As applies to sacroiliac joint fusion surgery
in 2017

(note that government oversite,
board of examiners, and surgical education societies did not
make it on the list)

Illustration two

**Entities considered most important in our healthcare
system today. The patient, who once was of highest
consideration and around which the entire medical
system revolved, has now fallen from the top of the
pyramid, to its lowest level, and least important position.**

The major difference in these two illustrations is that the "patient" is moved from the position of "most important" to a position of "least important".

How did this paradigm shift come about, and why? Concerning surgery for the SIJoint it started with the device industry's manipulation of the FDA 510(k) designation. This industry had recognized a need, designed and produced products to fill that need, launched new companies, found a way to circumvent the FDA, trained surgeons how to insert these new devices, created vast public awareness, and ultimately ended up with a very lucrative and continually increasing number of sacroiliac joint fusions being performed each passing year. It should be noted again that each of these devices is billed, on the average, at $10,000. The push to sell these implements began to impact what should have been of ultimate concern, the patient's welfare.

What the makers of these new devices did not emphasize is that they are capable of inflicting great harm if not inserted properly. Many significant problems have been reported, including severe hemorrhage, paralysis from nerve injuries, and pelvic bone fractures. In these instances, more surgeries have to be performed to resolve these complications. Therefore, it would seem to make sense that all involved participants should be rallying to first identify these issues, then research and develop improvements and solutions.

A good example of how a coordinated effort such as this could work to the patient's advantage was the development and implementation of another orthopedic device used to help fusions of the low back or lumbar spine. It is called the "pedicle screw," and is literally a screw inserted into what we call the "pedicle" of a vertebrae or spinal bone to serve as an anchor to which a rod can be attached. By doing this at multiple levels on the spine from the back, in the two pedicles located on each side of every level, long sections can be stabilized to achieve a boney fusion **(Figs. 10,11).**

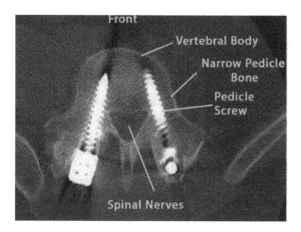

Fig 10.

CT scan cross-sectional view of one vertebral bone in the low back and the placement of pedicle screws within it. This makes for very solid and stable fixation points. Note that the nerves are just one or two millimeters away from the screw.

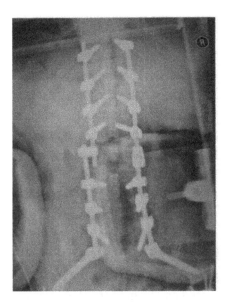

Fig 11.

X-Ray of multiple pedicle screws inserted into the bones of the spine, with rods attached, realigning the spine and holding it rigidly in place.

This segmental screw fixation originated in France, but was introduced in America during the late 1980s and early 90s. The one main difference between the pedicle screw and other fusion devices was that it was created *after* the formation of the FDA, meaning it was subjected to review and testing before being approved.

The pedicle screw, even when inserted properly, was and still is a valuable asset in achieving a solid spinal fusion. However, it is far from benign. If the screw is placed just a few millimeters off its intended course the first piece of anatomy it runs into is a spinal nerve, which can result in varying degrees of severe leg pain and even partial paralysis. If inserted too deeply, it can penetrate large blood vessels, which in some cases have resulted in death. During the early stages of use, its main regulating force was the legal profession, with thousands of lawsuits filed on behalf of patients suffering residual injuries. Most of the suits were aimed directly at the manufacturers, who put them into the hands of poorly trained surgeons. When the FDA stepped in to begin regulating the pedicle screw, it was deemed a "Class III device" (capable of causing paralysis or death).

Through a coordinated effort orchestrated at the highest levels of the surgical spine societies, and with the North American Spine Society (NASS) leading the way, surgeons, industry and the educational system went to work analyzing specific problems with the pedicle screw, creating solutions in design insertion techniques, developing sweeping educational reforms for surgeons, and making the pedicle screw a research priority by funding future clinical and laboratory studies.

Some of the outcomes from this emphasis on safety and education were that better educated and trained surgeons learned how to select patients most appropriate for this procedure. Complication rates also fell significantly. The FDA subsequently lowered the pedicle screw from "Class III" to "Class II", losing its designated potential for paralysis or death. Not only did surgical medical societies step up, but the American Board of Orthopedic Examiners added this procedure to surgeons' exams, ensuring higher proficiency in fusion work. The manufacturing industry also benefited, as the demand for pedicle screws grew exponentially. Everyone involved in providing top-notch care for those suffering from spinal ailments and requiring fusion surgery jumped aboard the ship. In this instance, the patient was certainly kept at the top of the "Pyramid of Importance."

Such was not the case for fusion devices manufactured for sacroiliac joint fusions after 2008. The fact that the industry had developed new devices certainly helped patients. All the educational efforts aimed at both surgeons and patients about sacroiliac joint pain also had positive effects. And, when these implements are inserted into the right patient for the right reasons and performed in a technically correct way, they most often provide pain relief or resolution. All of this was favorable for SI Joint pain sufferers. But what if surgeons are not properly educated in determining which patients fit the profile for these surgeries, and are not trained in the technicalities of the surgeries themselves? What if they are not trained to both identify and to treat complications when they do happen? This is when the situation becomes downright dangerous!

It has always been assumed that a surgeon is thoroughly trained by the medical educational system and surgical societies to meet a high standard of care. This includes diagnosing a condition, providing conservative treatment first, matching the best surgical procedure to each individual, performing it properly, and being prepared for complications. In our current reality surgeons are not adequately schooled in all these necessary areas regarding fusion surgery for the sacroiliac joint. There is no standardized education available to teach surgeons about this diagnosis. Based on my own experience and that of many other spine surgeons with whom I've spoken, board certification exams in both orthopedics and neurosurgery still do not test for proficiency in treating this condition. Neither is there any government oversight for this type of surgery.

Becker's Spine Review cites a study from iData research suggesting that by the year 2020, 50,000 sacroiliac joint fusions might be performed yearly. This begs the following questions. Who is in charge of protecting the escalating number of patients having the surgery? Who is ensuring those with this condition are properly diagnosed and undergo conservative treatment prior to a surgical implantation? Who is responsible for surgeons being trained to understand the anatomy surrounding the sacroiliac joint, insert these new devices, and understand and treat potential complications that do occur?

The answer is the surgical device industry! Since the FDA has certified all devices inserted through the lateral approach under the 510(k) designation, it has no further regulatory authority over them. The industry and the surgeons using its devices are supposed to report adverse situations as they occur. But one lengthy article on how the 510(k) designations are actually working estimates that only six percent of the time are reports submitted **(ref 11)**.

Since 2008, the device industry has not only influenced how medicine is taught, it has also taken the leading role in determining how surgery for sacroiliac joint pain is addressed. At $10,000 a pop for one of these surgical devices, a conflict of interest seems clear. We are actually worse off than in the early 1990s, with the pedicle screw, as no one is overseeing education or regulation.

Although the industry is only doing what is expected of it in a democratic capitalistic society, where profit is the main goal, intangibles like morality, ethics, and even patient importance take a backseat.

Surgeons who have aligned themselves with the industry further propagate this by having a vested interest in what industry is manufacturing while they are also the ones responsible for teaching other surgeons at the highest academic levels. If they are only instructing other surgeons about one device and one approach because they have a financial stake in it, they are helping to grossly misrepresent the entire scope of surgery possible for fusing the sacroiliac joint, and this only serves to stagnate the whole surgical education process. By both surgeons and the large surgical educational societies maintaining this narrow and profit-centered point of view, the bigger picture is ignored, and those who suffer with sacroiliac joint pain remain under-served.

This book has three purposes, all directed at helping people enduring this type of chronic pain. The first is to inform them that this diagnosis has been around for a long time and there are many treatments, conservative and surgical, that do work. The second is to make them aware that the system from which they are trying to obtain pain relief is flawed, and largely functions to make a profit, putting patient concerns in the background. Lastly, by better understanding the first two points, the lay person can navigate through the system, acting as his or her own advocate. Learning the steps that can be taken with clinicians, surgeons and institutions will hopefully help them find an accurate diagnosis, proper treatment, and ultimately a cure or at least significant reduction of ongoing pain.

The next chapter defines exactly what these steps are and how to accomplish them.

Being Your Own Advocate
Lessons on how America treats chronic sacroiliac joint pain

1 There is a 15-22% chance that your new chronic low back pain might be coming from your sacroiliac joint.

2 There is a high likelihood that your primary care doctor (except osteopaths), orthopedic surgeon, orthopedic spine surgeon, or neurosurgeon will not check you for a potential sacroiliac joint source of pain.

3 PTs, chiropractors and pain doctors are very good at diagnosing your dysfunctional sacroiliac joint, but they do not perform surgery. If you feel that the conservative treatments you are receiving for your pain are not curing the pain, but subjecting you to "endless treatments", you need to start looking for a surgical consultation. PTs have, in my experience, been the most helpful in this regard.

4 The only "Gold Standard" for accurately diagnosing your chronically painful sacroiliac joint is by an injection using X-Ray imaging, dye, and a long acting numbing medication, performed by a doctor trained in this procedure.

5 Currently word of mouth from patients and the Internet are your only options for seeking out surgical answers for your chronic sacroiliac joint pain as there exists no formal education for surgeons on this subject. Industry, which manufactures the very expensive devices for these fusions, is the current primary educator for surgeons. Keep in mind that until the formal educational teaching entities, such as medical schools and surgical societies, get on board and provide complete non-propriety training to surgeons concerning all aspects of treating the chronic disabling painful sacroiliac joint, the Internet will continue to harbor both solid and fruitful advice as well as many self-serving proprietary recommendations.

Chapter 8
The Sacroiliac Joint Playbook
How to confirm a dysfunctional sacroiliac joint diagnosis and steps for seeking treatment.

How does someone suffering with chronic low back pain find out if they might have a dysfunctional sacroiliac joint, and, if so, what do they do next? We need to invoke some garden-variety science and anatomy to answer this question.

If we start with the supposition that everything offered thus far has a semblance of truth to it, then one can assume that just going to the neighborhood immediate care center probably won't fly. If someone is indeed suffering from a chronically painful sacroiliac joint, knowing how to navigate the medical system can spare some of the frustration, discouragement, and emotional toll this process can often take. The following points provide basic information and key steps to consider before beginning this process.

1. Patient Advocates

There are two groups of clinicians who advocate for their patients with chronic sacroiliac joint pain not relieved by conventional therapies. They are the physical therapist and the primary care doctor. Physical therapists are trained in the diagnosis and manual treatment of the chronically painful sacroiliac joint. They are however, limited in their ability to provide treatment as they are only allowed by health insurance providers to treat a patient with a given diagnosis for a specified time period. If patients continue to have severe pain after this treatment period, they usually start looking for other solutions. Most physical therapists are willing to consult with a surgeon who has an interest in this condition. The primary care doctor can be an advocate, and is often encouraged by the physical therapist to make a referral to a surgeon. Some doctors, of course, care enough to look deeper and take the time to find an interested surgeon themselves.

2. Anatomy - Where is this joint anyway?

Everyone has two sacroiliac joints. They are located in the posterior of the pelvis. If someone reaches behind them to the top and middle of the groove between the buttocks, and with one-finger moves about 2 inches to one side and up another two inches, they feel a hard rounded boney mass. This is the area of the sacroiliac joint, with the joint located two to three inches deep from back to front. Its twin is on the opposite side in the same place. These two joints, along with the "pubic symphysis," (the bone in front of the pelvis that one can feel just above the genitals), comprise the three joints which hold the entire pelvic bone together. They are also the joints of the pelvic ring through which a baby's head passes during birth **(Fig 1).** The sacroiliac joints are a connection point where the sacrum (lowest segment of the entire spine) and the large winged iliac bones of the pelvis, one on each side, join together. All the forces from a person's head, arms and trunk transfer through these joints into the pelvis and directly into the hips and legs. Located right in the center of the body pain- free stability in the sacroiliac joints is crucial for nearly every type of daily activity.

3. Symptoms

One reason the sacroiliac joint is considered the "chameleon" of pain generators in the low back is the sheer number of ways it can present itself. Symptoms of a dysfunctional sacroiliac joint can be anything from an occasional ache to pain greater than that experienced during a vaginal delivery. The pain can be intermittent or constant, but the one thing that applies in all cases is that it can be exacerbated by normal activities. These include standing, standing on the leg on the same side as the sacroiliac joint, sitting, lying down on either side, walking, bending and lifting. The symptom that brings most sexually active women into a clinic is "dyspareunia," or painful intercourse. Men with a dysfunctional sacroiliac joint also describe a severe increase in back and pelvic pain accompanying thrusting movements during intercourse. The unique position of both sacroiliac joints, directly in the middle of the body at the level of the buttocks from front to back and side to side, enables them to generate pain to the back, the front, and down the back and front of the legs. Pain can occur in one or more of these areas. A clinician examining a patient can easily confuse this pain with that from a herniated lumbar disc or severe hip joint arthritis. If the pain is above and lateral from the top of the buttocks' groove, the sacroiliac joint is possibly the cause, or one of the causes.

4. Conservative Treatment

Patients beginning any course of conservative treatments should be informed about exactly what are considered appropriate methods, and how long they should take. At the time of this writing only one publication on this subject exists which has not been developed by an industrial company selling a device to fuse this joint. This published algorithm, or method, addresses appropriate conservative treatment for chronic sacroiliac joint pain, and can be found in **Appendix One** at the end of this book. I created this treatment method, along with how to appropriately diagnose this condition, through an evolutionary process while treating hundreds of patients with chronic low back pain from the sacroiliac joint.

The latest version of this algorithm along with an in-depth discussion of each step can be found in the textbook, Surgery *for the Painful Sacroiliac Joint: A Clinical Guide*, published in 2015 by Springer Publishing **(ref 6)**. This book is currently the only non-industry generated material available to orthopedic and neurosurgeons for treating the dysfunctional sacroiliac joint conservatively or surgically.

Steps for Finding Relief from Chronic Sacroiliac Joint Pain

Step 1. The History of Injury

First, a clinician should obtain a complete history as to how the patient's pain began. The elements that should alert them to a diagnosis of potential sacroiliac joint pain could include a fall, possibly from a height, with direct impact on the side or back of the pelvis, or an auto accident involving a head-on collision where the driver slammed on the brake with an outstretched straight leg resulting in back pain on that side. Another traumatic event could include the onset of low back and pelvic pain following a vaginal birth. Some more slowly developing causes for chronic sacroiliac joint pain could be a previous lumbosacral fusion with no pain resolution or the slow beginning of a new and lower back pain, a history of inflammatory arthritis associated with severe episodes of low back and pelvic pain, and a history of a short leg, pelvic tilting, or scoliosis (curvature of the spine). Keep in mind that the onset of pain in this joint can be insidious, with no history to account for when or how the pain began. Often, to quote many patients, "It just started one day."

Step 2. The Fortin Finger Test

Clinically, the single most valuable sign that should force a clinician to look at the sacroiliac joint as a possible pain generator, is the positive "Fortin Finger Test". Dr. Fortin discovered that when a patient reaches back and puts a finger on the spot just to the side of the groove or crack between the buttocks, and up directly on the rounded boney prominence, which we call the posterior superior iliac spine, the sacroiliac joint must be considered as the possible pain source. This test is illustrated in **Fig 6** of this book. If pain is also radiating from points higher up, the spine too must be considered. We have found that in almost half of sacroiliac patients diagnosed by injections, the lumbar spine is also a frequent co-pain generator. This would suggest, in order for all pain to be eliminated, that both areas need to be addressed. Here's where our present medical and surgical educational system falls terribly short. The training and experience of an average spine surgeon, whether an orthopedic or neurosurgeon, doesn't currently cover how to deal with this combination of pain generators. They typically address one, most likely the spine, and ignore the other. This is why many back surgeries can fail. Therefore, the message to someone hurting both at this boney prominence and a bit higher up in the low back, is that they need to be asking if they might have pain generators in the sacroiliac joint and the lumbar spine, as well as how each will be treated. If the answer is anything other than a confident and knowledgeable response, it may be advisable to look elsewhere for diagnosis and treatment.

Step 3.   First Type of Treatment

Once the sacroiliac joint is determined to be a possible pain source, assuming the patient has pain that has not been treated before, the first action is to treat it like garden-variety low back pain coming from any muscle or skeletal source. This can include anti-inflammatory medication, a sacral belt to provide support, and restriction of the activities that make the pain worse. Many patients will find significant relief just from these simple measures.

Step 4.   The Need for X-Rays

If the pain continues or worsens during this interval, X-Rays should be taken to illuminate other serious issues like tumors, infections, stress fractures, hip problems and a slew of other pathological conditions that require further treatment not part of this algorithm. The clinician should perform X-Rays during the first visit if certain "red flags" show up, which they have been trained to look for, suggesting that something other than an acute or chronic sacroiliac joint condition is causing the pain.

Step 5.   Manipulation of the Joint

The next step, with this now being a chronic problem, is to consider manipulation. Even though chiropractors rarely send sacroiliac joint patients to a qualified surgeon for definitive treatment, if I saw these patients first, I would always send them to a chiropractor before contemplating surgery. I learned early on that their manipulation processes on the sacroiliac joint frequently kept patients off the operating table. If a patient continues to feel pain after a proper manipulation routine lasting no longer than six weeks, they would be advised to return to my office to discuss next steps.

Why does this type of manipulation work? No one knows for sure. Many believe that this "shock wave", generated by the vigorous thrusting movement, changes pain generators at a cellular level, resulting in relief.

Step 6.   Physical Therapy

Next, assuming pain is still present and disabling, would be formal physical therapy. As I've said, these clinicians are very good at diagnosing a chronically painful sacroiliac joint. I have performed sacroiliac joint fusion surgery on a number of physical therapists, and they usually diagnosed themselves. The essence of what the P.T. does is stabilize and strengthen the surrounding muscles of the joint in order to relieve direct stress and hopefully, pain. One problem therapists run into while doing this is there are only a few small muscles that actually cross this joint. Despite their and the patient's best efforts these small muscles can have a difficult time becoming reliable stabilizers. Because these methods are effective in many cases, they should be attempted. However, building up small muscles to do the work of big ones can take a lot of time, which leads to a second possible problem. The health insurance companies they have to work with allow only a limited amount of time for physical therapy, which often is not long enough to determine if it is working. Once insurance runs out, many failed patients have no choice but to go to or go back to a chiropractor or pain doctor, and often end up in that revolving door of ongoing medical treatment.

Step 7.   Injections

Having followed this series of steps until now there has been no need for a definitive diagnosis, as everything thus far can be done through clinical, or hands-on

evaluation. This approach up to now has not been able to solicit a "rock-solid" diagnosis, thus enter the injection part of the workup and treatment for the painful sacroiliac joint. At this stage moving forward becomes more invasive and more costly.

The purpose of injections for sacroiliac joint pain is two-fold. The first is to make a definitive diagnosis of the sacroiliac joint as the origin of the pain. The second is to actually treat, and potentially cure it. Two medications are combined in each injection. One is a numbing anesthetic solution, which lasts between one to three hours. The other is a steroid designed to decrease all biochemicals in the joint responsible for generating pain. If a patient is properly injected by a trained clinician with the aid of an X-Ray, and he or she experiences near total relief for at least two hours, the sacroiliac joint is confirmed as the pain generator. If the steroid works well, that patient might get weeks, or even months, of pain relief. Although it is not common, sometimes with only one or two injections a patient might obtain permanent relief.

Those who respond to each injection with short-term relief, but don't obtain a cure, find themselves in that never-ending regimen of injection therapy, from which they can't seem to exit. What the average person, and even some clinicians, doesn't realize is that with each injection some of the chemicals, or vehicles, as we refer to them that carry the steroids are deposited in the joint and slowly build up with every subsequent injection. This was part of my research during my spine fellowship. These deposited chemicals have the ability to increase the rate of degenerative changes and arthritis in the joint. My advice to patients is that if they are not cured after four injections, the treatment is not working, and, if continued, could hasten deterioration of the joint and possibly increase pain in the long run.

Step 8.   Alternative Treatments

Once all routine, conservative treatments have been tried and injections have provided a conclusive diagnosis, there are multiple alternative treatments to consider. These include acupuncture, prolotherapy, radio frequency ablation and injections of other substances like hyaluronic acid. I won't delve into these here, other than mentioning that their success rate, in my experience, is 50/50. When one of them does work, it typically works well. I always encourage my patients to research all options, according to their interest, but I would not recommend any one of them over another.

If nothing has proven effective, and alternative treatments have at least been considered, the only remaining option is surgery. After having persevered and navigated the complex and often frustrating system to this point, being considered for surgery is a defining moment for a patient.

Step 9. Issues patients who are offered a sacroiliac joint fusion should consider

As previously stated, there is no current standard for performing these operations as set forth by the formal medical educational entities. The lateral minimally invasive approach has become the "pseudo-standard" championed by industry using various implantable devices made by them to result in increased stability or fusion of the joint. This approach and the devices used are approved by the FDA, but only because surgeries like these were performed successfully, for other purposes, prior to the establishment of that agency in 1976. Patients should understand that neither the FDA nor any entity within the medical system oversees fusion surgery outcomes for the chronically painful sacroiliac joint. This makes it crucial for patients to develop an open and trusting relationship with their surgeon, so that they can feel comfortable asking how the surgeon became interested in treating pain in this joint, how he or she was trained for these surgeries, as well as how many have been performed and what the success rate has been. Patients being considered for sacroiliac joint fusion need to be aware that there many potential approaches to access the sacroiliac joint **(Fig 12).**

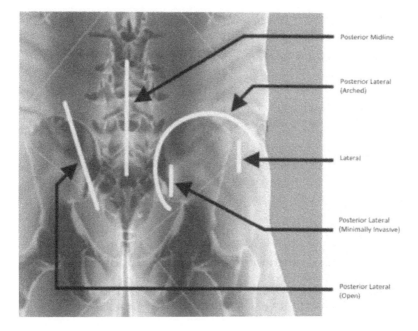

Posterior Midline

Posterior Lateral
(Arched)

Lateral

Posterior Lateral
(Minimally Invasive)

Posterior Lateral
(Open)

Fig 12. Diagram showing various incisions used to approach the sacroiliac joint from the back. Over the years there has been a movement toward more minimally invasive surgeries as evidenced by the shorter incisions. All the approaches shown average a 75% success rate for pain relief (ref 6).

Chapter 9
How To Be Your Own Advocate
Key questions to ask your pain doctor and surgeon.

Is the source of my pain my sacroiliac joint?

If your pain is the in the area the patient shown in **Fig 6** is pointing to, your clinician or surgeon needs to rule in or rule out the sacroiliac joint as a pain generator.

How is a painful dysfunctional sacroiliac joint diagnosed?

The standard for diagnosing a sacroiliac joint as a pain generator is by injection. This injection uses X-Ray imaging, places a needle into the base of the joint, and inserts a dye and anesthetic medication, along with a steroid. If a patient's pain is alleviated during the next 1 to 3 hours, the sacroiliac joint is determined to be a pain generator **(Fig 7).**

Who should I see for treatment of my chronically painful sacroiliac joint?

Consulting a physical therapist or chiropractor is a good start. Both are trained to diagnose and treat this condition. Although they may use different methods, they understand that the sacroiliac joint can cause pain. Many times they can significantly relieve or remove pain. If, after several weeks of treatment by a P.T. or chiropractor the pain is not resolved to a totally livable level, you should go to the next step.

Where should I go next if these conservative treatments fail?

A pain clinic is the next stop, as these are run by anesthesiologists and physiatrist who are highly trained to inject the sacroiliac joint with steroids in an effort to remove or significantly reduce pain permanently or for long intervals. Many times, they also try other modalities that might decrease or eliminate pain in the sacroiliac joint. These are referred to as "alternative treatments" and include prolotherapy, radio frequency ablation, cryotherapy, acupuncture and others.

What is my next option if injections and alternative treatments are not giving me the pain relief I need?

Surgery to fuse the sacroiliac joints together so they do not move is the only viable remaining option.

Who performs sacroiliac joint fusions?

Both orthopedic and neurosurgeons perform sacroiliac joint fusions. Here the burden is on the patient to seek out a surgeon who has an interest in treating this joint and is educated and trained in this area. Utilizing the Internet to find these surgeons is an option, as is word-of- mouth. At the time of this writing the best way to navigate the Internet is to do a search for "sacroiliac joint fusion" and look at the web sites that are not obviously sponsored by the device manufacturing industry. Once again, remember there is no formal educational structure for either orthopedic or neurosurgeons to diagnose or treat, either conservatively or surgically, the chronically painful sacroiliac joint. Surgeons with an interest in this have either learned on their own, have been trained by other self-taught surgeons, or have been educated by surgeons working for the industry selling devices to fuse this joint.

What are my options for how fusion surgery is performed and what are my chances for pain relief?

There are a number of approaches and devices for fusion surgery. With most of these, results for successfully relieving pain in the appropriate patient averages around 75%. The technique surgeons use is not as important as their knowledge of the anatomy involved and their surgical ability. The most common method used today is to insert industrially made devices across the sacroiliac joint from the side of the buttock in a minimally invasive fashion to stabilize or fuse it. Keep in mind that surgeons with a keen interest in surgically treating this joint may have devised methods or techniques for fusing this joint through their own "trial and error" methods over the years. Here it is important to understand how well their techniques worked in previous patients. It would be appropriate to ask your surgeon if you could speak with a patient that they had operated using their procedure.

What will my rehabilitation be like after I have surgery?

Located in **Appendix two** is an algorithm I created for industry to help the surgeons inserting their devices into patients understand a method for appropriate rehabilitation once the surgery is accomplished. Another resource is an excellent chapter written by Dr. Michael Rahl on the entire rehabilitation process after a successful sacroiliac joint fusion **(ref 6)**.

What are the most likely complications from the lateral minimally invasive approach with device insertion? (ref 12)

As with any surgery, complications may occur and should be thoroughly explained beforehand by your surgeon. Complications which are unique to the lateral approach   with device insertion include but are not limited to:

> a. Injury to large and small blood vessels
>
> b. Injury to large and small nerve structures
>
> c. Injury to the bowel

d. Fractures of the pelvis or sacrum

The above complications can result in additional surgery, which could comprise outcomes.

The medical literature states that these types of complications can occur between 1-17% of the time.

The very serious complications such as a pulmonary embolism, infection, a lasting morbidity and even death can occur with this surgery as with any major elective surgery. Most surgeons would state that the chances for such complications occurring are far less than 1%.

What are some questions regarding sacroiliac joint chronic pain and treatment for which we don't yet have definitive answers?

What is it within the sacroiliac joint that generates pain?

Are there certain specific movements of this joint that are more prone to generating pain?

What role exactly does arthritis play in causing or worsening sacroiliac joint pain, and why, when no obvious arthritis is present, can this joint still have severe pain?

Who are the best candidates for a sacroiliac joint fusion?

Which surgical approach is best for the patient?

Which fusion method works best in relieving sacroiliac joint pain?

What are the long-term effects on a patient undergoing fusion of one or both sacroiliac joints?

Should there be long-term limitations on activity after having one or both sacroiliac joints fused?

When pain generators are present in both the sacroiliac joints and the lumbar spine at the same time is it best to fuse one first then the other if needed, or both at the same time?

This list goes on and on, with many more questions currently unanswered. Having no active surgical society or government sponsored research attempting to find answers is of major concern, especially if *Becker's Spine Review* is correct in its estimation that by the year 2020, 50,000 of these surgeries will be performed annually in this country.

The knowledge base for the chronically painful sacroiliac joint is literally "stuck in the mud" in America today. After a century of knowing how this joint can disrupt lives it is almost unbelievable that we don't know more! This is the time for the very individuals who are suffering with this pain to learn all they can and challenge our medical system for the needed answers. Only this way can we move forward together in such a way as to keep the patient at the top of the pyramid in the place of "most important".

Chapter 10
Epilogue

This book is the culmination of my work with the painful sacroiliac joint over the past three decades, consisting of conservative treatment, surgical intervention and laboratory cadaver research. It also includes the experiences of several other surgeons who I have met on my journey and who have also been involved with the mysteries and frustration of this joint. Much of this book results from the experiences of my patients, who have suffered with this condition, and became their own advocates by seeking help to relieve their pain. Most have undergone various types of sacroiliac joint fusion surgery, were rehabilitated back to a functional state, and went on to give back by donating their personal medical data and experience for research and publication purposes, as well as counseling others with the same condition. In my mind these early patients are true pioneers in our medical system's attempt to further understand the pain these joints can cause and how to go about properly treating them, both conservatively and surgically.

It would be easy to look at entrepreneurial surgeons, hospitals for profit, industrialists selling devices for a king's ransom and the medical educational societies, who are influenced by financial contributions from the medical manufacturing industry, as the "Evil Empire," but that would be fruitless. America is a free democratic capitalistic society. And all four of these entities, each impacting the sacroiliac patient, are doing what is expected of them within this system. Unfortunately, the main ingredient in patient care that continues to recede is compassion, which then leads to a loss of basic human ethics. This is where patients who suffer with a chronically painful sacroiliac joint have not been adequately diagnosed or cared for. These patients must make a considerable effort to learn about their condition and find surgeons who are knowledgeable and caring. This is not an easy task in the U.S., where current forces seem to make it an uphill battle. However, armed with some basic knowledge, experience of others, and some intestinal fortitude, lasting pain relief is a hopeful and reasonable goal for anyone suffering with chronically painful and disabling sacroiliac joints.

One more comment is in order, and that is to briefly discuss what the future holds for those suffering from this disabling and chronic condition. In short, these four key players in the medical system, outlined above, are going to have any options for surgical treatment locked up for the indefinite future. This means there will be one type of surgery available, using one of the 510k designated devices, and will take place with absolutely no oversight from the FDA, surgical medical educational societies, or surgeon proficiency examining boards. I am not saying that this is all bad; the system seems to be helping many patients, but the average person can readily see that options are limited and many of the complications and pitfalls that do happen are kept under the radar.

There is, however, a grassroots effort taking place to move forward, though it is not located in America. It is centered in Europe, by a group of orthopedic and neurosurgeons who come together each year to discuss current knowledge about fusing the sacroiliac joint, different ways of approaching it, and the many devices which can be used to assist a surgeon in successfully completing a fusion. They also review potential complications along with ways to deal with them, and the results of on-going research. None of this is happening in our country today that is not influenced by the medical technology industry. The European organization is called SIMEG (Sacroiliac Medical Expert Group). Here, surgeons, industry and educational societies are working together, with the primary goal of finding answers to the many unresolved issues relating to SI Joint pain, and how to provide the highest levels of care and treatment. They are light years ahead of us. The United States could be approaching the future of the sacroiliac joint in the same way as our European friends, but it would take a tremendous paradigm shift to accomplish that. We would need to understand how a patient is looked upon in a capitalistic health care system versus one which views patient health as an inalienable right, and whose medical system includes healthcare payment for these surgeries. In this country, our hope is that someday we will not only learn from the European healthcare system, but actually put into practice what it has already been doing for years.

About the Author

Bruce Dall was born in South Omaha. He attended the University of Nebraska Medical Center, Michigan State University's affiliated orthopedic residency program and Southern Illinois University's spine fellowship. He became an orthopedic spinal surgeon in 1985 and began his practice at Borgess Medical Center in Kalamazoo, Michigan. As a young, highly educated, but by his own admission, a yet naive surgeon who expected to have all the answers, Dr. Dall soon realized he, along with his peers, knew little to nothing about how the sacroiliac joint related to chronic back pain, as it was not receiving any attention from the medical education establishment. He also learned that countless patients were suffering from chronic back pain which traditional treatments often failed to relieve. He then began a quest for answers about how to diagnose and treat chronic sacroiliac joint problems, now proven to be a prime generator for back pain.

Dr. Dall's research and self-training led him to literally create his own treatments, including surgery, for patients whose suffering from chronic sacroiliac joint pain had not been relieved by antiquated and poorly understood textbook methods.

The sources for this book include Dr. Dall's thirty years' experience in the diagnosis and treatment of hundreds of patients with chronic sacroiliac joint pain, as well as the shared experiences of several colleagues, laboratory research, and a century's worth of literature on the subject of fusing the sacroiliac joints together when all other treatment methods failed. He has published several clinical studies on long-term outcomes from surgeries. His development of a minimally invasive method to fuse sacroiliac joints was published in a peer reviewed journal in 2008, and his production of an algorithm to guide clinicians and surgeons through this diagnosis was published as a white paper in 2010.

Following this, the Borgess Brain and Spine Institute, where he practiced from 2005 to 2013, became not only a national referral source for chronic sacroiliac pain, but began receiving inquiries from patients in countries around the world.

In collaboration with the few other orthopedic spine surgeons in America who understood and shared his interest, he created a textbook for surgeons and physical therapists, *Surgery for the Painful and Dysfunctional Sacroiliac Joint: a clinical guide,* on how to diagnose and treat sacroiliac joint pain patients, which was published by Springer Publishing Company in November 2014. The following year he published a paper in a peer-reviewed orthopedic surgical journal about patients who suffered from both pain in the lumbar spine and the sacroiliac joint at the same time; the first study to discuss performing a fusion on both areas in one setting.

Currently, Dr. Dall is an Associate Professor at Western Michigan University School of Medicine. He is involved in ongoing clinical and laboratory research on the sacroiliac joint, and continues to write on the subject for medical professionals and those suffering from chronic sacroiliac joint pain.

Disclosure: Dr. Dall has no vested interest in any device being manufactured or sold by industry for the purpose of fusing the sacroiliac joint.

Disclaimer: The contents of this book are considered to be for general educational purposes only and are in no way meant to be construed as medical treatment. The author claims no responsibility for any adverse outcomes that might result from anyone following the advice given in this book. Before deciding to commit to any form of treatment, conservative or surgical, each individual should consult with his or her doctor.

References

1. Zelle BA, Gruen GS, Brown S, George S. Sacroiliac joint dysfunction: evaluation and management. Clin J Pain. 2005; 21: 446-55.

2. Bernard TN, Kirkaldy-Willis WH. Recognizing specific characteristics of non-specific low back pain. Clin Orthopedic. 1987; 217: 266-80.

3. Schwarzer AC, Aprill CN, Bogduk N. The sacroiliac joint in low back pain. Spine. 1995; 20: 31-7.

4. Smith-Petersen MN, Rogers WA. End-result study of arthrodesis of the sacroiliac joint for arthritis-traumatic and non-traumatic. J Bone Joint Surgery Am. 1926; 8: 118-36.

5. Dall, B.E., Priest, B.; A Clinical Marker for Premenopausal Osteoporosis: Hypermobility of the Second Metacarpalphalangeal Joint, Today's Therapeutic Trends: The Journal of New Developments in Clinical Medicine, Volume 10, Number 1, pages 22-37, 1992.

6. Dall BE, Eden SV, Rahl MD. Surgery for the Painful Dysfunctional Sacroiliac Joint: A Clinical Guide, Springer Publishing, International, print ISBN: 978-3-319-10725-7; e-book ISBN:978-3-319-10726-4. http://www.springer.com/us/book/9783319107257

7. Dall BE, Eden SV. Outcomes of bilateral sacroiliac joint fusions and the importance of understanding potential coexisting lumbosacral pathology that might also require surgical treatment. Acta Orthop Belg. 2015, 81, 233-239.

8. Fortin JD, Falco FJ. The Fortin Finger Test: an indicator of sacroiliac pain. Am J Orthop. 1997 Jul; 26 (7): 477-480.

9. Maine JY, Aivaliklis A, Pfefer F. Results of the sacroiliac joint double block and value of sacroiliac provocation tests in 54 patients with low back pain. Spine. 1996; 21: 1889-92.

10. Beckers Spine Review: http://www.beckersspine.com/spine/item/23039-si-joint-fusion-could-explode-by-2020-5-things-

11. Sorenson C. Drummond M. Improving Medical Device Regulation: The United States and Europe in Perspective. Milbank Q. 2014 Mar; 92(1): 114-150. Doi: 10.1111/1468-0009.12043

12. Rudolf L. Open Orthop J. 2013 May 17; 7:163-8. doi: 10.2174/1874325001307010163.
PMID: 23730380 Free PMC Article
(Many of the complications that do occur with the lateral minimally invasive approach to fuse this joint are discussed in this often referenced article.)

APPENDIX ONE

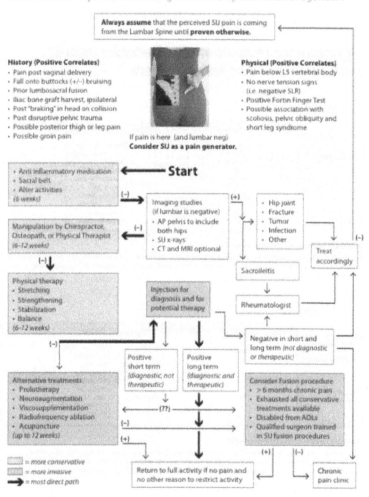

Sacroiliac Joint Dysfunction: A Borgess Brain & Spine Institute Algorithm

Always assume that the perceived SIJ pain is coming from the Lumbar Spine until proven otherwise.

History (Positive Correlates)
- Pain post vaginal delivery
- Fall onto buttocks (+/−) bruising
- Prior lumbosacral fusion
- Iliac bone graft harvest, ipsilateral
- Post "braking" in head on collision
- Post disruptive pelvic trauma
- Possible posterior thigh or leg pain
- Possible groin pain

If pain is here (and lumbar neg)
Consider SIJ as a pain generator.

Physical (Positive Correlates)
- Pain below L5 vertebral body
- No nerve tension signs (i.e. negative SLR)
- Positive Fortin Finger Test
- Possible association with scoliosis, pelvic obliquity and short leg syndrome

Start

- Anti inflammatory medication
- Sacral belt
- Alter activities
  (6 weeks)

Manipulation by Chiropractor, Osteopath, or Physical Therapist
(6-12 weeks)

Physical therapy
- Stretching
- Strengthening
- Stabilization
- Balance
  (6-12 weeks)

Alternative treatments
- Prolotherapy
- Neuroaugmentation
- Viscosupplementation
- Radiofrequency ablation
- Acupuncture
  (up to 12 weeks)

Imaging studies
(if lumbar is negative)
- AP pelvis to include both hips
- SIJ x-rays
- CT and MRI optional

- Hip joint
- Fracture
- Tumor
- Infection
- Other

Treat accordingly

Sacroileitis

Injection for diagnosis and for potential therapy

Rheumatologist

Negative in short and long term (not *diagnostic or therapeutic*)

Positive short term (*diagnostic, not therapeutic*)

Positive long term (*diagnostic and therapeutic*)

Consider Fusion procedure
- > 6 months chronic pain
- Exhausted all conservative treatments available
- Disabled from ADLs
- Qualified surgeon trained in SIJ fusion procedures

(??)

Return to full activity if no pain and no other reason to restrict activity

Chronic pain clinic

▨ = more conservative
▨ = more invasive
➤ = most direct path

APPENDIX TWO

(Authored by Bruce E Dall, MD and provided as a courtesy of ZYGA Corporation. Please see Dr. Dall's disclaimer in Preface.)

Algorithm for Post-operative Rehabilitation of the Sacroiliac Joint fusion Patient

0-6 Weeks

	Bracing	Amb assist	Weight-bearing	Lifting	Therapy	Avoid
In-joint Approach	SI Belt when up. Not needed in shower	Crutches or walker for 3 weeks, then discard	Can set foot on floor bearing up to 20#. After 3 weeks, full weight-bearing using short stride.	Up to 15#	**Aquatic:** Core muscle strengthening and gait and/or **Land:** Core muscle strengthening, active (only) muscle stretching, ambulation and ADLs (all using biomechanically correct techniques)	Bending or twisting at the waist at all times
Out-of-joint Approach		Crutches or walker	Toe touch only			
Obese, Either Approach	Ineffective	Walker	Can set foot on floor bearing up to 20#			

Suggested PT prescription for 0-6 weeks post-op:

Water therapy for gradual active muscle stretching and core muscle strengthening. Work on balance, gait and essential ADLs. Use only biomechanically appropriate bending at the waist. No lifting more than 15#. Avoid manual pressure techniques. Can use modalities PRN. May transition to land during this time if patient demonstrates appropriate capability.

6-12 Weeks

	Bracing	Amb assist	Weight-bearing	Lifting	Therapy	Avoid
In-joint Approach		None		From 15# to full (slow increase with increasing strength of associated musculature)	**Land:** Core muscle strengthening, stabilizing, strengthening and balancing long and large pelvic, trunk and associated extremity musculature.	Bending or twisting at the waist at all times
Out-of-joint Approach	No brace needed		Full weight-bearing using shorter stride			
Obese, Either Approach	-	Walker				

Suggested PT prescription for 6-12 weeks post-op:

Core strengthening. Stabilization, strengthening and balancing of the major and long muscle groups involving the pelvic, trunk and associated extremities. Use modalities PRN. Perfect gait and abilities to perform all ADLs using biomechanically correct techniques. Teach home exercise and stretching program reinforcing above. Avoid inappropriate bending and twisting at waist. Slowly progress to patient's full lifting capacity.

Other Books by this author:

Surgery for the painful dysfunctional sacroiliac joint: a clinical guide

Dall, Eden & Rahl editors
Copyright 2015
Springer Publishing Company
http://www.springer.com/
us/book/9783319107257

Lightning Source UK Ltd.
Milton Keynes UK
UKHW021842151118
332415UK00020B/637/P